KETOGENIC DIET + ELECTRIC PRESSURE COOKER

Box set

100 Easy Recipes for Healthy Eating, Healthy Living & Weight Loss

Modern Kitchen

I

TABLE OF CONTENTS

KETOGENIC DIET

50 Easy Recipes for Healthy Eating, Healthy Living & Weight Loss

Modern Kitchen

INTRODUCTION TO KETOGENIC DIET

This book contains helpful facts about the ketogenic diet. It will help you understand the basics and benefits of the diet. It has simple steps and tips to get you through the diet. It also contains tasty and easy-to-do keto recipes you'll enjoy.

History of the Ketogenic Diet

The use of fasting to treat certain diseases, including epilepsy, can be traced to the physicians of ancient times. But because prolonged fasting often results in muscle loss and nutrient deficiencies, doctors eventually began to study modified diets. During the early 1920s, Dr. Russel Wilder developed the ketogenic diet and used it to treat epileptics. It remained a popular treatment for epilepsy, especially in children, through the next decade. But when improved anticonvulsant medications were developed around 1940, the use of ketogenic diets declined.

In 1994, the ketogenic diet regained its popularity thanks to Charlie Abrahams, a boy who suffered from epilepsy despite using anticonvulsant medications and other medical treatments. His seizures were controlled only through the implementation of the ketogenic diet. This inspired his father, Hollywood producer Jim Abrahams, to set up the Charlie Foundation, which promotes and funds research about the diet. Since then, further studies have been made, and less restrictive models have become available for people seeking general health improvement and also for those desiring weight loss.

Mechanism of the Ketogenic Diet

A typical modern diet is high in carbohydrates. That causes the body to use glucose as its primary source of energy. Fats, macronutrients that normally serve as an energy source, are therefore not used and are instead stored. On the other hand, the ketogenic diet's high-fat, moderate-protein, low-carbohydrate program causes the body to turn to fats as its energy source. Because of the lack of carbs, the liver will convert stored fats into ketone bodies and release them into the blood. These will then be used as fuel instead of the glucose from carbs. This metabolic state is called ketosis. When your body is in ketosis, fats are easily consumed rather than stored. That's why it is also called the "fat-burning mode" of the body. Ketosis is a normal result of staying on a low-carb diet (or of prolonged fasting or starvation).

Different enzymes are used for breaking down carbs and fats. Therefore, a body that is used to a high-carb diet will have to adjust before entering into ketosis. This may take three to four days. Before building up a new supply of enzymes, the body will first use up all the glucose that is left, resulting in weakness and lethargy. But once the body has adapted to ketosis, it will be able to maximize the use of fats. Some advocates of the keto diet even testify that they experience longer lasting energy throughout the day.

Is Ketosis dangerous?

Ketosis is often feared due to the confusion between it and ketoacidosis. If ketosis is the body's normal response to a low-carb diet, ketoacidosis is an abnormal condition where excessive ketone bodies in the bloodstream have overwhelmed the body's homeostasis – the compensatory mechanisms of the body – resulting in acidic blood pH. Ketosis is rumored to lead to ketoacidosis because ketone bodies are acidic. However, ketoacidosis actually results from a shortage of insulin, and is not due to a prolonged state of ketosis. So the only people at risk for ketoacidosis are those with type 1 diabetes or pancreatic disorders.

Food list

A keto diet is basically increasing your dietary fat intake, choosing low-carb foods, and avoiding high-carb foods. It should be at least 70% fat, around 25% protein, and only 5% carbohydrates. When choosing foods, pick those that are closest to their natural forms. As much as possible, choose raw over preserved foods, organic over highly processed, grass-fed or free-range over caged animals, wild caught over farmed fish, etc.

Below is a list of low-carb foods you can choose from:

Fats & oils

- Almond
- Avocado
- Butter
- Ghee
- Lard
- Olive
- Nut oils
- Seed oils
- Mayonnaise
- Peanut butter
- Cocoa butter
- Coconut
- Chicken fat
- Beef tallow
- Bacon fat

Note: Limit intake of oils rich in omega-6 fatty acids, such as nut oil, canola oil, corn oil, sunflower oil and margarine. Choose cold pressed vegetable oils.

Meat

- Beef
- Bacon
- Pork chops
- Lamb
- Veal
- Ham
- Goat
- Pork loin
- Wild game
- Sausage
- Chicken
- Duck
- Quail
- Goose
- Turkey
- Pheasant
- Any wild-caught fish or seafood

- Whole eggs

Note: Choose fattier cuts of meat from grass-fed or free-range animals.

Vegetables

- Asparagus
- Alfalfa
- Avocado
- Bell pepper
- Bamboo sprouts
- Brussels sprouts
- Beet greens
- Broccoli
- Bean sprouts
- Bok choy
- Celery
- Cabbage
- Carrots
- Chives
- Cucumber
- Cauliflower

- Chard
- Collard greens
- Leeks
- Radishes
- Onion
- Kale
- Garlic
- Spinach
- Scallions
- Tomatoes
- Snow peas
- Summer squash
- Shallot
- Water chestnut
- Turnip

Note: Avoid starchy veggies such as potatoes, winter squash, etc.

Nuts & seeds

- Almond
- Macadamia

- Walnut
- Pecan
- Cashew
- Chestnut
- Pistachio
- Any kind of seeds

Note: Nuts and seeds are high in omega-6 fatty acids and some have higher carb content, so it is best to limit intake. They are best consumed when soaked and roasted.

Dairy

- Whipping cream
- Sour cream
- Cream cheese
- Any kind of cheese
- Yogurt

Note: Choose full fat and organic dairy products.

Beverages

- Herbal tea
- Decaf coffee and tea

- Almond milk
- Soy milk
- Coconut milk
- Lime juice
- Lemon juice

Note: Choose unsweetened options.

Sweeteners

- Stevia
- Xylitol
- Monk fruit
- Lo han guo
- Chicory root
- Splenda
- Erythritol

Note: Choose liquid sweeteners over powdered ones.

Fruits

Berries such as blueberries, strawberries, etc.

Seasonings

Any low-carb spices without added sugar

Benefits of the Ketogenic Diet

Brain protection

The ketogenic diet was originally designed to treat epilepsy, a neurological disease characterized by recurrent and uncontrollable shaking or seizures. These seizures are caused by abnormal and excessive activities of the nerve cells in the brain. Epilepsy is now usually treated with anticonvulsant medications or surgery. But in some cases where such medications are ineffective, a ketogenic diet is implemented.

It is unclear how exactly the diet works, but in many cases it lessens the number of seizures by 50% or more, especially in children. Clinical trials show that ketone bodies have the capacity to protect brain cells from damage and prevent their premature death. They suggest that ketogenic diets can also prevent or reverse other neurodegenerative disorders such as Parkinson's and Alzheimer's. The use of the diet for this purpose is still in the research stage.

Heart health

Many people are skeptical about the ketogenic diet because of its high fat intake. They believe that fats increase cholesterol levels and clog the arteries. However, current studies dismiss this myth and actually prove that a ketogenic diet can be beneficial for the cardiovascular system.

Fats or lipids in the bloodstream can be found in two forms: triglycerides and cholesterol. A triglyceride is a fatty acid that stores energy, and cholesterol is a molecule used by the body to aid in absorption of vitamins, cell maintenance, hormone regulation, etc. This means that fat is essential for the body to function normally. Now, cholesterol is transported throughout the body in the blood by molecules called lipoproteins. These lipoproteins are classified depending on their density: low-density lipoproteins (LDL) and high-density lipoproteins (HDL).

HDL is known as the good cholesterol because it not only transports cholesterol, it also brings unused cholesterol back to the liver to be broken down. This prevents it from clogging the arteries and leading to cardiovascular disease. Thus, increased HDL is ideal for maintaining a healthy cardiovascular system. LDL, on the other hand, is commonly referred to as the bad cholesterol because it moves more slowly than HDL and has a tendency to clog arteries when oxidized by free radicals. LDL comes in different forms: the larger it is the better for you; the smaller and denser the form the more harmful it is.

One study shows that low-carb diets significantly increase the level of HDL cholesterol compared to low-fat diets. Another study suggests that low-carb diets can help reduce LDL levels and increase the size of LDL molecules. The ketogenic diet, therefore, is beneficial to your cardiovascular system as it helps increase the good HDL and decrease the bad LDL.

Weight loss

The most effective way to lose weight permanently is to deal with its root cause. There are many causes of weight gain, but the dominant one is hormonal imbalance. Overeating and living a sedentary lifestyle are obvious reasons for gaining weight; however, these are actually symptoms of a hormonal imbalance related to insulin, the hormone responsible for moving glucose into the cells to be used as fuel. When the body's insulin is abnormally high, it becomes dependent on glucose for fuel and refuses to use up stored fats. This is the underlying reason for overeating. And low energy levels, caused by the hormonal imbalance, hinder a more active lifestyle.

The main cause of increased insulin levels is high carbohydrate consumption, which is a common feature of an average diet. When glucose from carbs accumulates in the blood, the body releases more insulin in order to deal with it. Too much carb intake increases both levels of blood sugar and insulin. This will eventually lead to high blood pressure, weight gain and other related diseases.

In other words, the ketogenic diet is one of the best weight loss programs because it maintains normal levels of insulin, keeps hormones balanced and prevents any increase of blood sugar levels. You will feel fewer cravings, which helps prevent overeating; and you'll have higher energy levels for more activities that help you lose weight.

Summary

The purpose of the ketogenic diet is primarily for health improvement, but because of its weight loss benefits many dieters have joined the program. Fortunately, the keto diet plan is a healthy and easy way to lose those extra pounds. In a keto diet, counting calories is made easy and cooking meals made fun!

Thanks again for downloading this book, I hope you enjoy it!

Ok, onto the recipes...

Enjoy!

BREAKFAST

Almond-Pumpkin Smoothie

Ingredients

2 cups almond milk

1 cup pumpkin puree

1 tsp pure vanilla extract

½ cup water

ice cubes (optional)

cacao nibs (optional)

Instructions

1. Mix all the ingredients in a blender and pulse until silky smooth.

2. Serve in chilled glass and enjoy.

Servings: 3

Cooking Time: 5 minutes

Nutrition Facts

Serving size: 1/3 of a recipe (7.7 ounces)

Percent daily values based on the Reference Daily Intake (RDI) for a 2000 calorie diet.

Amount Per Serving

Calories 285.1

Calories From Fat (85%) 243.1

% Daily Value

Total Fat 29.0g 45%

Saturated Fat 25.7g 129%

Cholesterol 0mg 0%

Sodium 117.4mg 5%

Potassium 384.9mg 11%

Total Carbohydrates 7.3g 2%

Fiber 1.2g 5%

Sugar 1.5g

Protein 3.2g 6%

Curly Kale "Ice Cream" Shake

Ingredients

1 ½ cup curly green kale leaves

½ cup heavy (whipping) cream

½ cup filtered water

½ cup raw cashews

2 Tbsp liquid sweetener of your choice

1 tsp vanilla extract

1 tsp finely minced ginger

pinch of Celtic sea salt

ice cubes (optional)

Instructions

1. Throw all of the ingredients in your blender and puree until smooth and creamy. 2. Add ice cubes and enjoy your day!

Servings: 2

Preparation: 5 minutes

Nutrition Facts

Serving size: 1/2 of a recipe (7.7 ounces)

Percent daily values based on the Reference Daily Intake (RDI) for a 2000 calorie diet.

Amount Per Serving

Calories 141.2

Calories From Fat (50%) 69.9

% Daily Value

Total Fat 8.4g 13%

Saturated Fat 1.6g 8%

Cholesterol 0mg 0%

Sodium 28.6mg 1%

Potassium 390.2mg 11%

Total Carbohydrates 9.2g 3%

Fiber 2g 8%

Sugar 2.7g

Protein 4.5g 9%

Easy Lemon Poppy Seed Muffins

Ingredients

4 eggs

2 tsp poppy seeds

1 tsp sesame seeds

1 cup almond flour

4 Tbsp olive oil

½ cup sweetener of your choice

3 Tbsp lemon juice

1 tsp vanilla extract

½ tsp baking soda

zest of one lemon

salt

Instructions

1. Preheat oven to 320°F. Prepare 12 muffin cups.

2. Place all ingredients in your blender and mix well until smooth.

3. Divide batter evenly among the muffin cups. Bake for 30 minutes.

4. When ready, cool and serve.

Servings: 12

Cooking Time

Total Time: 40 minutes

Nutrition Facts

Serving size: 1/12 of a recipe (1.3 ounces)

Percent daily values based on the Reference Daily Intake (RDI) for a 2000 calorie diet.

Amount Per Serving

Calories 111.2

Calories From Fat (52%) 57.3

% Daily Value

Total Fat 6.5g 10%

Saturated Fat 4.7g 24%

Cholesterol 47.1mg 16%

Sodium 71.4mg 3%

Potassium 49.7mg 1%

Total Carbohydrates 8.4g 2%

Fiber 0.5g 2%

Sugar 2.7g

Protein 2.9g 6%

Homemade Energetic Bar

Ingredients

1 cup almonds

¼ cup pecans

1 cup peanuts

1 cup shredded coconut

1 cup almond butter

1 cup coconut oil, freshly melted and still warm

4 Tbsp sweetener of your choice (optional)

1 Tbsp chocolate chips (optional)

Instructions

1. Place the almonds, pecans, peanuts in a food processor and chop them for 1 to 2 minutes.

2. Add in the shredded coconut, almond butter, sweetener and coconut oil. Process for one minute.

3. Place parchment paper on a square container and place the mixture on top.

4. Whisk the mixture vigorously, with a spatula and then with the hand.

5. Place the chocolate chips on top and press them slightly with your hands.

6. Place the container in the freezer for 3 to 4 hours.

7. Remove from the freezer and cut into rectangular pieces with a large knife.

8. Serve.

Servings: 8

Nutrition Facts

Serving size: 1/8 of a recipe (1.3 ounces)

Amount Per Serving

Calories 223.4

Calories From Fat (78%) 174.6

% Daily Value

Total Fat 20.7g 32%

Saturated Fat 8.6g 43%

Cholesterol 0mg 0%

Sodium 32.4mg 1%

Potassium 163.5mg 5%

Total Carbohydrates 8.2g 3%

Fiber 2.8g 11%

Sugar 3.3g

Protein 4.5g 9%

Mediterranean Mint and Feta Omelette

Ingredients

3 eggs

6 fresh mint leaves

4 ounces feta cheese

salt and freshly ground black pepper, to taste

olive oil

Instructions

1. In bowl, beat eggs with feta cheese and chopped fresh mint. Season salt and pepper. Mix well.

2. In a frying pan add olive oil and pour the egg mixture; cook over medium to high heat for 2 to 3 minutes.

3. With the wooden spoon turn the omelette to other side and cook one minute more.

4. When done, the bottom will be set and the edges will look crisp.

5. Transfer omelette to a plate and serve hot. Enjoy!

Servings: 2

Cooking Time

Total Time: 15 minutes

Nutrition Facts

Serving size: 1/2 of a recipe (2.8 ounces)

Percent daily values based on the Reference Daily Intake (RDI) for a 2000 calorie diet.

Amount Per Serving

Calories 113.7

Calories From Fat (60%) 68.1

% Daily Value

Total Fat 7.6g 12%

Saturated Fat 2.6g 13%

Cholesterol 279.9mg 93%

Sodium 259.7mg 11%

Potassium 113.2mg 3%

Total Carbohydrates 0.8g <1%

Fiber 0.1g <1%

Sugar 0.3g

Protein 9.9g 20%

Nutty Eggs with Avocado

Ingredients

4 large eggs

½ avocado, sliced

½ cup walnuts, sliced

2 Tbsp olive oil

½ tsp cilantro (optional)

sea salt and freshly ground black pepper to taste

Instructions

1. Heat the oil in a skillet over medium-high heat.

2. Beat the eggs in a small bowl and pour into the skillet.

3. Cook for 1 minute and turn heat to medium-low. Cook about 3 minutes more.

4. Top with walnuts, avocado and cilantro.

5. Season with sea salt and freshly ground black pepper to taste.

6. Serve.

Servings: 2

Nutrition Facts

Serving size: 1/2 of a recipe (5.1 ounces)

Percent daily values based on the Reference Daily Intake (RDI) for a 2000 calorie diet.

Amount Per Serving

Calories 286.5

Calories From Fat (73%) 208.8

% Daily Value

Total Fat 24.5g 38%

Saturated Fat 4.1g 20%

Cholesterol 247.4mg 82%

Sodium 194.5mg 8%

Potassium 438mg 13%

Total Carbohydrates 7.6g 3%

Fiber 4.4g 18%

Sugar 1.3g

Protein 2.1g 24%

Pancake Torte with Ham and Bacon

Ingredients

6 keto pancakes

4 slices of bacon

4 slices ham

2 cups shredded cheddar cheese

fresh parsley (chopped)

coconut oil

Instructions

1. Top one keto pancake with one slice of bacon, ham, parsley and shredded cheese.

2. Place another pancake on top of the filling and repeat the procedure.

3. Continue until you finish with all bacon, ham and cheese.

4. Cook in frying pan on medium-low heat with coconut oil, and cover with a lid until the cheese is melted.

5. Flip and cook 1-2 minutes on the other side.

6. Let cool. Cut and serve hot.

Servings: 8

Cooking Time

Preparation Time: 25 minutes

Nutrition Facts

Serving size: 1/8 of a recipe (3.5 ounces)

Percent daily values based on the Reference Daily Intake (RDI) for a 2000 calorie diet.

Amount Per Serving

Calories 314.1

Calories From Fat (66%) 207.7

% Daily Value

Total Fat 23.3g 36%

Saturated Fat 10.8g 54%

Cholesterol 74.7mg 25%

Sodium 737.1mg 31%

Potassium 168.7mg 5%

Total Carbohydrates 8.6g 3%

Fiber 0g 0%

Sugar 0.2g

Protein 16.9g 34%

Vegetable Omelette

Ingredients

3 eggs

1 medium zucchini

1 green onion (white and green parts), chopped

1 green pepper

2 tsp parmesan cheese – grated

2 cloves garlic

Salt and ground black pepper to taste

Instructions

1. Wash and dry all vegetables and dice finely.

2. Heat frying pan with the olive oil and sauté the garlic, green onion and pepper about 5 minutes. Add salt and pepper to taste.

3. Add the diced zucchini, stir and cook 3-4 minutes more.

4. In a bowl, beat the eggs with parmesan cheese.

5. Pour egg mixture over the vegetables and cook for 3 minutes per side.

6. Serve hot.

Servings: 3

Cooking Time

Total Time: 35 minutes

Nutrition Facts

Serving size: 1/3 of a recipe (10.6 ounces)

Percent daily values based on the Reference Daily Intake (RDI) for a 2000 calorie diet.

Amount Per Serving

Calories 128.4

Calories From Fat (37%) 47.4

% Daily Value

Total Fat 5.3g 8%

Saturated Fat 1.7g 8%

Cholesterol 186mg 62%

Sodium 84.4mg 4%

Potassium 614.2mg 18%

Total Carbohydrates 9.7g 4%

Fiber 3.3g 13%

Sugar 7.2g

Protein 8.9g 18%

LUNCH

Baked Pickled Cabbage with Ham

Ingredients

14 oz ham

3 green onions, chopped

2 bay leaves

1 head pickled cabbage

4 cloves garlic (chopped)

2 dry red peppers

a few peppercorns

4 Tbsp oil

salt & black pepper to taste

Instructions

1. Preheat oven to 400°F.

2. Cut the ham into pieces and put in a saucepan with water; bring to boil.

3. Add the onion (cut in half or in quarters), bay leaf and a few peppercorns.

4. Cook about 30 minutes.

5. Remove the ham and set aside on a plate.

6. Chop the onion, leek and dry red paprika.

7. In a separate bowl, finely chop the pickled cabbage.

8. Heat the large frying pan with oil, add the onion and chopped dried peppers, and stir well.

9. Add the cabbage and cook about 30 minutes over medium heat, stirring constantly. Adjust salt and ground black pepper to taste. Remove from the fire.

10. In a greased baking dish put half of the fried cabbage, layer with the ham, and cover with the remaining cabbage.

11. Pour just enough water to cover the cabbage.

12. Bake in the oven for about 1 hour. Serve hot.

Servings: 8

Cooking Time

Total Time: 2 hours

Nutrition Facts

Serving size: 1/8 of a recipe (9 ounces).

Percent daily values based on the Reference Daily Intake (RDI) for a 2000 calorie diet.

Amount Per Serving

Calories 174.5

Calories From Fat (42%) 72.9

% Daily Value

Total Fat 8.2g 13%

Saturated Fat 1.6g 8%

Cholesterol 11mg 4%

Sodium 480.6mg 20%

Potassium 437.7mg 13%

Total Carbohydrates 15.7g 5%

Fiber 4.8g 19%

Sugar 6.8g

Protein 11.5g 23%

Beef, Asparagus and Mushroom Stew

Ingredients

1 ¼ lb beef filets

½ lb mushrooms, thinly sliced

1 cup asparagus, cooked and cut into small pieces

2 cloves garlic

2 green onions, finely chopped

½ cup bell pepper (green or red)

1 tsp minced garlic

pinch of turmeric

2 Tbsp olive oil

½ tsp dried rosemary

Salt and freshly ground black pepper to taste

Instructions

1. Add the oil in an oven-proof skillet. Add in the onion, red pepper, and garlic and sauté 2-3 minutes.

2. Add mushrooms and cook for two to three minutes more. Stir in rosemary, salt and pepper to taste.

3. In medium bowl, combine the onion mixture with asparagus and beef chunks and set aside.

4. In a greased frying skillet over medium-high heat, cook meat and the vegetable mixture.

5. Reduce heat to medium-low and cook 10 to 15 minutes.

6. Serve hot.

Servings: 6

Cooking Time

Total Time: 35 minutes

Nutrition Facts

Serving size: 1/6 of a recipe (7.5 ounces)

Percent daily values based on the Reference Daily Intake (RDI) for a 2000 calorie diet.

Amount Per Serving

Calories 315.4

Calories From Fat (71%) 222.5

% Daily Value

Total Fat 24.3g 37%

Saturated Fat 8.5g 43%

Cholesterol 70.9mg 24%

Sodium 69.9mg 3%

Potassium 521.2mg 15%

Total Carbohydrates 5g 2%

Fiber 1.9g 8%

Sugar 2.3g

Protein 19.3g 39%

Cashews Chicken and Watercress Stir-Fry

Ingredients

1 ¼ lb beef filets

½ lb mushrooms, thinly sliced

1 cup asparagus, cooked and cut into small pieces

2 cloves garlic

2 green onions, finely chopped

½ cup bell pepper (green or red)

1 tsp minced garlic

pinch of turmeric

2 Tbsp olive oil

½ tsp dried rosemary

Salt and freshly ground black pepper to taste

Instructions

1. Add the oil in an oven-proof skillet. Add in the onion, red pepper, and garlic and sauté 2-3 minutes.

2. Add mushrooms and cook for two to three minutes more. Stir in rosemary, salt and pepper to taste.

3. In medium bowl, combine the onion mixture with asparagus and beef chunks and set aside.

4. In a greased frying skillet over medium-high heat, cook meat and the vegetable mixture.

5. Reduce heat to medium-low and cook 10 to 15 minutes.

6. Serve hot.

Servings: 6

Cooking Time

Total Time: 35 minutes

Nutrition Facts

Serving size: 1/6 of a recipe (7.5 ounces)

Percent daily values based on the Reference Daily Intake (RDI) for a 2000 calorie diet.

Amount Per Serving

Calories 315.4

Calories From Fat (71%) 222.5

% Daily Value

Total Fat 24.3g 37%

Saturated Fat 8.5g 43%

Cholesterol 70.9mg 24%

Sodium 69.9mg 3%

Potassium 521.2mg 15%

Total Carbohydrates 5g 2%

Fiber 1.9g 8%

Sugar 2.3g

Protein 19.3g 39%

Creamy Zucchini and Broccoli Soup

Ingredients

2 leeks (white part only)

4 big green zucchinis

1 cup broccoli (shredded)

3 Tbsp virgin olive oil

5 cups water

Salt and black pepper, to taste

Parmesan cheese – grated

Instructions

1. Heat the olive oil in a large saucepan, and add the chopped leeks.

2. Cook the leeks until soft (8-10 minutes), stirring gently.

3. Add the chopped zucchini and broccoli and sauté about 5 minutes.

4. Add water, bring to a boil and simmer without covering for about 15-17 minutes.

5. Process the soup in batches until smooth.

6. Ladle to plates, sprinkle with grated cheese and serve.

Servings: 4

Cooking Time

Total Time: 45 minutes

Nutrition Facts

Serving size: 1/4 of a recipe (15.7 ounces).

Percent daily values based on the Reference Daily Intake (RDI) for a 2000 calorie diet.

Amount Per Serving

Calories 74.9

Calories From Fat (9%) 6.6

% Daily Value

Total Fat 0.8g 1%

Saturated Fat 0.2g <1%

Cholesterol 0mg 0%

Sodium 176.4mg 7%

Potassium 672.4mg 19%

Total Carbohydrates 11.7g 5%

Fiber 3.2g 13%

Sugar 5.0g

Protein 3.4g 7%

Curry Broccoli Cream Soup

Ingredients

1 ¼ lb broccoli

1 cup cauliflower florets

2 green onions (green parts only, minced)

2 white celery stalks

3 Tbsp olive oil

1 onion

3 cups water

curry to taste

ginger

salt and pepper (to taste)

splash of cream or evaporated milk

Instructions

1. In a saucepan or pot with oil, sauté chopped green onion and celery.

2. Add in the broccoli and cauliflower.

3. Add the curry, ground ginger and salt and pepper to taste.

4. Pour in water to cover the vegetables. Bring to boil and cook 10-12 minutes over low heat.

5. Once everything is cooked through, place in a blender, add a splash of cream or evaporated milk, and blend until smooth.

6. Adjust salt to taste and serve.

Servings: 4

Cooking Time

Total Time: 40 minutes

Nutrition Facts

Serving size: 1/4 of a recipe (10.9 ounces)

Percent daily values based on the Reference Daily Intake (RDI) for a 2000 calorie diet.

Amount Per Serving

Calories 164.4

Calories From Fat (56%) 91.2

% Daily Value

Total Fat 10.3g 16%

Saturated Fat 1.4g 7%

Cholesterol 0mg 0%

Sodium 18.5mg <1%

Potassium 321.3mg 9%

Total Carbohydrates 11.2g 6%

Fiber 2.3g 9%

Sugar 3.4g

Protein 1.9g 4%

Keto Grilled Shrimps

Ingredients

14 ounces fresh shrimp

2 Tbsp olive oil

sea-salt flakes

rosemary sprig, leaves finely chopped

Instructions

1. Rinse the whole shrimp and then drain them.

2. Heat some oil on a grill pan. Place shrimp on grill and cook 5-7 minutes, turning halfway through the process.

3. The outside of the shrimp should turn a nice pink color when it is cooked.

4. Place shrimp on the serving plate and sprinkle with sea-salt flakes.

5. Serve.

Servings: 2

Cooking Time

Total Time: 30 minutes

Nutrition Facts

Serving size: 1/2 of a recipe (7.6 ounces)

Percent daily values based on the Reference Daily Intake (RDI) for a 2000 calorie diet.

Amount Per Serving

Calories 119.3

Calories From Fat (91%) 101.3

% Daily Value

Total Fat 13.5g 21%

Saturated Fat 1.9g 9%

Cholesterol 0mg 0%

Sodium 0.3mg <1%

Potassium 0.1mg <1%

Total Carbohydrates 0g 0%

Fiber 0g 0%

Sugar 0g

Protein 0g 0%

Lemony Grilled Chicken

Ingredients

3 lbs chicken breast

5 limes or lemons, sliced

1 tsp allspice

1 Tbsp onion powder

1 Tbsp smoked paprika

1 Tbsp garlic powder

sea salt and freshly ground black pepper to taste

Instructions

1. Prepare your barbecue grill.

2. In a large bowl, place chicken pieces and lemon rings.

3. In a small bowl, combine paprika, onion powder, garlic powder, allspice, salt and pepper to taste.

4. Pour the spice mixture over chicken and mix thoroughly.

5. Grill chicken and lemon rings on barbecue over medium heat for 10-12 minutes per side.

6. Sprinkle with chopped parsley and serve hot.

Servings: 6

Cooking Time

Total Time: 45 minutes

Nutrition Facts

Serving size: 1/6 of a recipe (11.3 ounces)

Percent daily values based on the Reference Daily Intake (RDI) for a 2000 calorie diet.

Amount Per Serving

Calories 289.9

Calories From Fat (19%) 55.6

% Daily Value

Total Fat 6.3g 10%

Saturated Fat 1.4g 7%

Cholesterol 145.2mg 48%

Sodium 268.6mg 11%

Potassium 1029.4mg 29%

Total Carbohydrates 9.6g 4%

Fiber 5.0g 20%

Sugar 0.2g

Protein 29.8g 50%

Mackerel Fish and Shrimp Soup (Slow Cooker)

Ingredients

1 lb mackerel fish fillets

2 cups frozen shrimp

1 cup cauliflower florets

½ cup carrots

1 cup zucchini (medium, sliced)

½ green onion finely chopped

heart of celery

2 cloves garlic

1 cup heavy whipping cream

3 cups water

salt and fresh ground pepper to taste

Instructions

1. Chop up the vegetables.

2. Cube the fish and dump everything (except the cream and the shrimp) into your slow cooker.

3. Cover and cook on LOW for 8-10 hours.

4. About 30 minutes before serving, stir in your cup of cream and the frozen shrimp.

5. Turn your slow cooker to HIGH for the last 30 minutes.

6. Serve hot.

Servings: 6

Cooking Time

Total Time: 9 hours

Nutrition Facts

Serving size: 1/6 of a recipe (9.3 ounces)

Percent daily values based on the Reference Daily Intake (RDI) for a 2000 calorie diet.

Amount Per Serving

Calories 235.3

Calories From Fat (63%) 147.8

% Daily Value

Total Fat 16.8g 26%

Saturated Fat 9.7g 48%

Cholesterol 84.9mg 28%

Sodium 288mg 12%

Potassium 266.9mg 8%

Total Carbohydrates 3.7g 1%

Fiber 0.6g 2%

Sugar 0.9g

Protein 17.4g 35%

Savory Belgian Endives Salad with Cheddar

Ingredients

4 Belgian endives

2 oz cheddar cheese, cut into small cubes

3 Tbsp fresh parsley leaves, coarsely chopped

3 Tbsp fresh lemon juice

3 Tbsp of olive oil

Salt and pepper to taste

Instructions

1. Cut and remove the bottom of the endives and wash in cold water.

2. In a bowl, whisk well the olive oil, lemon juice and salt and pepper to taste.

3. Place endives in a salad bowl and add the cheddar cheese cubes and the chopped parsley.

4. Sprinkle with lemon juice dressing, toss the salad, and serve immediately.

Servings: 4

Cooking Time

Total Time: 15 minutes

Nutrition Facts

Serving size: 1/4 of a recipe (6.9 ounces)

Percent daily values based on the Reference Daily Intake (RDI) for a 2000 calorie diet.

Amount Per Serving

Calories 150.2

Calories From Fat (87%) 131.3

% Daily Value

Total Fat 14.9g 23%

Saturated Fat 4.4g 22%

Cholesterol 14.9mg 5%

Sodium 89.9mg 4%

Potassium 41.6mg 1%

Total Carbohydrates 1.2g <1%

Fiber 0.13g <1%

Sugar 0.4g

Protein 3.7g 7%

DINNER

Avocados Stuffed with Shrimp

Ingredients

2 cups small shrimp, cooked and washed

4 large avocados

1 Tbsp lemon juice

2 Tbsp fresh cilantro

2 Tbsp mayonnaise

1 Tbsp onion powder

1 tsp black pepper

1 Tbsp paprika

Salt to taste

Instructions

1. Put the avocados on a plate with the cut side up.

2. In a medium bowl, mix the shrimp, lemon juice, fresh cilantro, onion and pepper. Place the shrimp mixture in each avocado, covering generously.

3. Pour the mayonnaise over stuffed avocados. Serve immediately.

Servings: 6

Nutrition Facts

Serving size: 1/6 of a recipe (5.6 ounces)

Percent daily values based on the Reference Daily Intake (RDI) for a 2000 calorie diet.

Amount Per Serving

Calories 222.1

Calories From Fat (74%) 165.2

% Daily Value

Total Fat 19.6g 30%

Saturated Fat 2.7g 14%

Cholesterol 3.8mg 1%

Sodium 57-96mg 2%

Potassium 640.0mg 18%

Total Carbohydrates 10.1g 4%

Fiber 8.6g 34%

Sugar 0.9g

Protein 2.9g 6%

Chilled Cauliflower and Cilantro Soup

Ingredients

1 lb cauliflower

½ can (11 oz) coconut milk

½ cup water

½ tsp fresh ginger

3 sprigs fresh cilantro

2 Tbsp olive oil

Salt and pepper to taste

Instructions

1. Place the cauliflower in a large pot and cover with water.

2. Bring to a boil over high heat, then reduce heat to medium-low, cover, and simmer 5 to 7 minutes.

3. Remove from heat, drain and let cool several minutes.

4. Put the cauliflower in a bowl and beat together with the coconut milk.

5. While beating, add the water little by little until you get the desired texture.

6. With a mortar, crush the ginger and cilantro and add to the cauliflower.

7. Beat again to combine all the ingredients.

8. Serve cold.

Servings: 4

Nutrition Facts

Serving size: 1/4 of a recipe (4.4 ounces).

Percent daily values based on the Reference Daily Intake (RDI) for a 2000 calorie diet.

Amount Per Serving

Calories 120.8

Calories From Fat (93%) 111.9

% Daily Value

Total Fat 13g 20%

Saturated Fat 6.5g 32%

Cholesterol 0mg 0%

Sodium 5.4mg <1%

Potassium 77.9mg 2%

Total Carbohydrates 1.8g <1%

Fiber 0.0g <1%

Sugar 0.0g

Protein 0.5g 1%

Ground Beef and Kale Stew with Cashews

Ingredients

1 Tbsp coconut oil

1 lb ground beef

2 cups curly kale

1 tsp ground cumin

1 tsp oregano

1 tsp garlic powder

salt and freshly ground black pepper, to taste

1 cup cashews

Instructions

1. In a pan, melt the coconut oil and cook the beef over medium heat.

2. Browning ground beef should take approximately 7 to 10 minutes for 1 pound of meat.

3. Add the cumin, oregano, garlic powder, ground pepper and salt; stir.

4. Add chopped kale and cook for 5 minutes.

5. Remove from the heat, sprinkle with chopped cashews and serve.

Servings: 4

Nutrition Facts

Serving size: 1/4 of a recipe (7.2 ounces)

Percent daily values based on the Reference Daily Intake (RDI) for a 2000 calorie diet.

Amount Per Serving

Calories 397.6

Calories From Fat (74%) 412.5

% Daily Value

Total Fat 35.8g 59%

Saturated Fat 19.6g 98%

Cholesterol 150mg 50%

Sodium 138.8mg 6%

Potassium 536.0mg 15%

Total Carbohydrates 0.7g <1%

Fiber 0.2g <1%

Sugar 0.0g

Protein 35.5g 71%

Kale Broccoli Cream Soup

Ingredients

1 ¾ lb broccoli

2 scalions, chopped

2 celery stalks, chopped

1 ½ cups kale (finely chopped)

ginger

curry to taste

3 Tbsp olive oil (or butter)

water

Instructions

1. Heat the oil in a pot; sauté chopped green onion and celery 1 to 2 minutes.

2. Add in the broccoli and kale. Add salt and pepper to taste, and add in the curry and ground ginger.

3. Pour water to cover vegetables, cover and boil for 4 to 5 minutes, until tender.

4. Once everything is cooked through, beat until a very thin consistency is reached and add a splash of cream or evaporated milk.

5. Adjust salt and pepper and serve.

Servings: 4

Cooking Time

Total Time: 40 minutes

Nutrition Facts

Serving size: 1/4 of a recipe (7.2 ounces).

Percent daily values based on the Reference Daily Intake (RDI) for a 2000 calorie diet.

Amount Per Serving

Calories 173.5

Calories From Fat (53%) 91.5

% Daily Value

Total Fat 10.4g 16%

Saturated Fat 1.4g 7%

Cholesterol 0mg 0%

Sodium 31.4mg 1%

Potassium 430.6mg 12%

Total Carbohydrates 11.0g 4%

Fiber 2.7g 11%

Sugar 2.7g

Protein 2.2g 4%

Salmon Ratatouille

Ingredients

1 lb salmon

1 scallion, roughly chopped

1 green pepper

1 eggplant

1 zucchini

3 Tbsp extra virgin olive oil

½ cup water

1 tsp sweet pepper powder

pepper & salt to taste

dill

granulated garlic

Instructions

1. Preheat oven to 400°F.

2. In a frying pan with olive oil, sauté chopped eggplant and zucchini 3 to 4 minutes.

3. Add in chopped scallion and green pepper.

4. Cover; cook over medium-low heat, stirring often, for 7 to 10 minutes, or until eggplant is tender.

5. Pour the water, cover and cook for an additional 20 minutes.

6. Add in one teaspoon of sweet pepper powder. Adjust salt and pepper.

7. Spread the aluminium paper over your working surface. Share the vegetable mixture among three or four aluminium pieces.

8. Place the salmon over the vegetables and close the wrap.

9. Place the salmon wraps in the oven and bake for 15-17 minutes.

10. Serve hot.

Servings: 4

Cooking Time

Total Time: 55 minutes

Nutrition Facts

Serving size: 1/4 of a recipe (9.3 ounces).

Percent daily values based on the Reference Daily Intake (RDI) for a 2000 calorie diet.

Amount Per Serving

Calories 80.2

Calories From Fat (5%) 4.1

% Daily Value

Total Fat 0.5g <1%

Saturated Fat 0.1g <1%

Cholesterol 0.1mg <1%

Sodium 15.2mg <1%

Potassium 527.5mg 15%

Total Carbohydrates 9.4g 4%

Fiber 5.6g 22%

Sugar 5.4g

Protein 2.5g 5%

Slow Cooker Beef Soup

Ingredients

1 ½ lbs round steak

1 cup scallion, roughly chopped

2 cups water

1 cup sweet potato, peeled and cut into cubes

1 carrot, sliced thinly

4 Tbsp lemon juice

salt and pepper, to taste

2 Tbsp olive oil

Instructions

1. Add beef strips to the bottom of your slow cooker.

2. Add the oil, chopped scallions, carrots and sweet potato.

3. Pour in water, cover and cook on LOW 6 to 8 hours.

4. Serve hot.

Servings: 6

Cooking Time

Total Time: 8 hours

Nutrition Facts

Serving size: 1/6 of a recipe (9.1 ounces)

Percent daily values based on the Reference Daily Intake (RDI) for a 2000 calorie diet.

Amount Per Serving

Calories 282.4

Calories From Fat (59%) 167.1

% Daily Value

Total Fat 18.6g 29%

Saturated Fat 5.6g 28%

Cholesterol 70.3mg 23%

Sodium 95.6mg 4%

Potassium 534.1mg 15%

Total Carbohydrates 7.6g 3%

Fiber 1.5g 6%

Sugar 2.2g

Protein 20.6g 41%

Spinach Almond Purée

Ingredients

1 lb fresh spinach (well washed)

2 cups cauliflower florets

2 green onions (white and green parts), chopped

4 Tbsp olive oil

4 cups water

¼ cup roasted almonds, chopped

Instructions

1. Wash, clean and cut all vegetables.

2. In a non-stick frying pan, fry the almonds 2-3 minutes; remove from the heat and set aside.

3. Heat the olive oil in a deep pan and cook the cauliflower and green onion for about two minutes.

4. Add the cleaned spinach leaves, water and salt to taste. Bring to a boil and let it simmer for 15 minutes.

5. Remove from the heat and place the vegetables in a food processor along with some toasted almonds. Blend until smooth.

6. Ladle purée into bowls and serve.

Servings: 4

Cooking Time

Total Time: 45 minutes

Nutrition Facts

Serving size: 1/4 of a recipe (13.4 ounces)

Amount Per Serving

Calories 72.4

Calories From Fat (36%) 26.0

% Daily Value

Total Fat 3.1g 5%

Saturated Fat 0.3g 2%

Cholesterol 0mg 0%

Sodium 122.2mg 5%

Potassium 906.1mg 26%

Total Carbohydrates 8.7g 3%

Fiber 4.6g 18%

Sugar 1.9g

Protein 5.7g 11%

Stuffed Portobello Mushrooms

Ingredients

8 large Portobello mushrooms

2 leeks

1 spring onion (medium-large)

1 green pepper

2 Tbsp cream

4 Tbsp parmesan cheese

salt and pepper to taste

Instructions

1. Preheat oven to 350°F.

2. Clean the mushrooms with a damp paper towel. Remove the stems and cut in half.

3. Cut the green and hard part of the leeks. Cut in half lengthwise and wash

4. well under a stream of water, opening the leaves to remove any dirt. Cut into thin slices.

5. Wash and remove the stalks and white parts of the peppers; chop into cubes.

6. In a large skillet heat 1 tablespoon vegetable oil or butter over medium heat and cook the leeks, stirring about 5 minutes.

7. Add the chopped vegetables and cook about 3-4 more minutes, stirring occasionally. Season with salt and pepper to taste.

8. Add the cream and turn off the heat; stir until incorporated well.

9. Place the mushrooms in a greased baking pan and season with salt.

10. Stuff every mushroom with the vegetable mixture and sprinkle with parmesan cheese.

11. Bake in oven for 25 minutes.

12. Serve hot.

Servings: 8

Cooking Time

Total Time: 55 minutes

Nutrition Facts

Serving size: 1/8 of a recipe (7.5 ounces)

Percent daily values based on the Reference Daily Intake (RDI) for a 2000 calorie diet.

Amount Per Serving

Calories 85.2

Calories From Fat (30%) 25.2

% Daily Value

Total Fat 2.9g 4%

Saturated Fat 1.5g 7%

Cholesterol 7.0mg 2%

Sodium 116.9mg 5%

Potassium 675.0mg 19%

Total Carbohydrates 10.8g 4%

Fiber 2.9g 11%

Sugar 4.4g

Protein 6.4g 13%

Sweet Potato and Spinach Tortilla

Ingredients

1 ¼ cup grated sweet potato

6 eggs (preferably organic)

2 cups spinach

1 Tbsp olive oil

1 green onion, diced

2 Tbsp minced parsley

salt to taste

Instructions

1. In a large bowl beat the eggs and combine with chopped parsley. Set aside.

2. Heat the olive oil in a frying pan and sauté the onion and the sweet potatoes.

3. Season with salt; cook over medium heat for 5 minutes, stirring occasionally.

4. Add the spinach and cook for another 1 minute.

5. Add this mixture to the eggs and mix well.

6. Pour the egg and spinach mixture in the pan and cook for 3 minutes per side over medium heat.

7. Serve hot.

Servings: 4

Cooking Time

Total Time: 30 minutes

Nutrition Facts

Serving size: 1/4 of a recipe (7.7 ounces)

Percent daily values based on the Reference Daily Intake (RDI) for a 2000 calorie diet.

Amount Per Serving

Calories 138.5

Calories From Fat (58%) 80.0

% Daily Value

Total Fat 8.9g 14%

Saturated Fat 2.6g 13%

Cholesterol 279mg 93%

Sodium 193.3mg 8%

Potassium 242.4mg 7%

Total Carbohydrates 4.1g 1%

Fiber 0.9g 4%

Sugar 1.7g

Protein 10.2g 20%

SNACKS

Absolute Avocado Pizza

Ingredients

dough

2 eggs

4 Tbsp grated cheese

2 envelopes unflavored gelatin

1/2 cup sour cream

4 Tbsp water

3 Tbsp butter

salt to taste

fresh parsley (chopped)

filling: ham, bacon, cheddar / mozzarella cheese, mushrooms, avocado puree (instead of tomato sauce)

Instructions

1. Preheat oven to 450°F.

2. Place all ingredients in a blender (without dissolving the gelatin) and beat well.

3. Grease parchment paper with butter and evenly distribute the dough.

5. Place in greased baking pan and bake about 15 minutes.

6. Remove pizza from the oven and spread evenly with avocado sauce.

7. Top with ham, bacon, fresh parsley and mushrooms and sprinkle with the cheese.

8. Bake for 5-10 minutes.

9. Remove from oven, slice and serve immediately.

Servings: 4

Cooking Time

Total Time: 30 minutes

Nutrition Facts

Serving size: 1/4 of a recipe (5.7 ounces)

Percent daily values based on the Reference Daily Intake (RDI) for a 2000 calorie diet.

Amount Per Serving

Calories 267.7

Calories From Fat (69%) 184.6

% Daily Value

Total Fat 20.87g 32%

Saturated Fat 11.4g 57%

Cholesterol 162.8mg 54%

Sodium 800.1mg 33%

Potassium 242.0mg 7%

Total Carbohydrates 1.2g <1%

Fiber 0g 0%

Sugar 0.2g

Protein 18.3g 37%

Baked Parsnip Fingers

Ingredients

2 parsnips, sliced

2 Tbsp olive oil

salt to taste

Instructions

1. Preheat oven to 350°F.

2. Wash, peel and cut the parsnip in sticks. Season with salt to taste.

3. Line a baking pan with parchment paper and toss olive oil over it.

5. Place in oven and bake about 10-12 minutes until golden brown.

6. Serve hot or cold.

Servings: 6

Cooking Time

Total Time: 20 minutes

Nutrition Facts

Serving size: 1/6 of a recipe (3.3 ounces)

Percent daily values based on the Reference Daily Intake (RDI) for a 2000 calorie diet.

Amount Per Serving

Calories 106.5

Calories From Fat (39%) 42.0

% Daily Value

Total Fat 4.8g 7%

Saturated Fat 0.7g 3%

Cholesterol 0mg 0%

Sodium 9.0mg <1%

Potassium 333.8mg 10%

Total Carbohydrates 10.0g 4%

Fiber 4.4g 17%

Sugar 4.3g

Protein 1.1g 2%

Flaxee Eggplant Dip

Ingredients

3 medium eggplants, peeled

6 Tbsp flaxseed flour

1 Tbsp extra virgin olive oil

2 cloves garlic

1 green onion, chopped

1 cup light mayonnaise

salt to taste

water

Instructions

1. Place eggplant, chopped green onion, garlic, water and salt in a pot and bring to a boil.

2. Cover and cook over medium heat for 12-13 minutes, or until eggplant cubes are cooked and soft.

3. Drain in a strainer and allow to cool.

4. Remove from heat and add flaxseed meal. Add the mayonnaise until a smooth paste forms.

5. Serve with your favorite keto crackers.

Servings: 8

Cooking Time

Total Time: 25 minutes

Nutrition Facts

Serving size: 1/8 of a recipe (3.4 ounces)

Percent daily values based on the Reference Daily Intake (RDI) for a 2000 calorie diet.

Amount Per Serving

Calories 122.4

Calories From Fat (85%) 104.3

% Daily Value

Total Fat 11.6g 18%

Saturated Fat 1.7g 9%

Cholesterol 10.5mg 4%

Sodium 240.0mg 10%

Potassium 40.9mg 1%

Total Carbohydrates 4.2g 1%

Fiber 0.3g 1%

Sugar 1.9g

Protein 0.4g <1%

Italiano Fat Balls

Ingredients

1 cup cream cheese

7 slices bacon

¼ cup green olives, pitted and chopped

2 Tbsp fresh basil, chopped

2 Tbsp pesto sauce

1 tsp fresh parsley, chopped

salt and pepper to taste

Instructions

1. Slice pitted olives and the bacon into small pieces.

2. In a bowl, mix together cream cheese, basil and pesto.

3. Add the olives and bacon into the cream cheese and mix again. Add fresh parsley. Mix well.

4. Form into 6 balls and serve immediately.

5. Keep refrigerated

Servings: 6

Cooking Time

Total Time: 10 minutes

Nutrition Facts

Serving size: 1/6 of a recipe (3.4 ounces)

Percent daily values based on the Reference Daily Intake (RDI) for a 2000 calorie diet.

Amount Per Serving

Calories 370.6

Calories From Fat (87%) 322.5

% Daily Value

Total Fat 36.2g 56%

Saturated Fat 14.8g 74%

Cholesterol 74.1mg 25%

Sodium 577.8mg 24%

Potassium 203.5mg 6%

Total Carbohydrates 3.3g 1%

Fiber 0.8g 3%

Sugar 1.3g

Protein 8.7g 17%

Peppermint Artichoke Hearts

Ingredients

6 artichoke hearts with stems, row trimmed

4 cloves garlic, minced

3 cups water

4 Tbsp extra-virgin olive oil

3 Tbsp fresh peppermint leaves, chopped

3 Tbsp fresh cilantro leaves, chopped

2 Tbsp fresh lemon juice

Salt and freshly ground black pepper, to taste

Instructions

1. In a deep pan, place artichokes along with water, oil, cilantro leaves, peppermint, lemon juice, and garlic.

2. Season with salt and pepper to taste and bring to a boil. Reduce heat and simmer artichokes about 15–20 minutes, turning occasionally.

3. Transfer artichokes to a serving platter and drizzle with some of the cooking liquid.

4. Serve.

Servings: 4

Nutrition Facts

Serving size: 1/4 of a recipe (12.8 ounces)

Percent daily values based on the Reference Daily Intake (RDI) for a 2000 calorie diet.

Amount Per Serving

Calories 201.3

Calories From Fat (60%) 121.4

% Daily Value

Total Fat 13.8g 21%

Saturated Fat 1.9g 9%

Cholesterol 0mg 0%

Sodium 149.1mg 6%

Potassium 559.6mg 16%

Total Carbohydrates 11.5g 5%

Fiber 8.3g 33%

Sugar 0.2g

Protein 5.5g 11%

Raw Pistachio Flaxseed Burgers

Ingredients

½ cup ground flaxseed

1 cup pistachio

4 cloves garlic

2 Tbsp lemon juice

2 Tbsp olive oil

sea salt to taste

Instructions

1. Place all ingredients in a food processor; process until well blended.

2. Form two patties with your hands.

3. Serve immediately or refrigerate patties for several hours.

Servings: 3

Cooking Time

Total Time: 15 minutes

Nutrition Facts

Serving size: 1/3 of a recipe (3.7 ounces)

Percent daily values based on the Reference Daily Intake (RDI) for a 2000 calorie diet.

Amount Per Serving

Calories 318.2

Calories From Fat (74%) 235.6

% Daily Value

Total Fat 27.7g 43%

Saturated Fat 3.5g 18%

Cholesterol 0mg 0%

Sodium 1.4mg <1%

Potassium 446.9mg 13%

Total Carbohydrates 13.3g 4%

Fiber 4.3g 17%

Sugar 3.4g

Protein 8.7 g 17%

Olive Crackers with Rosemary

Ingredients

¼ cup chia seeds

½ cup whole flaxseeds

1 large egg

1 egg white

2 sprigs fresh rosemary (cleaned from the steam)

4 Tbsp extra virgin olive oil

sea salt

1 cup of water

Instructions

1. Preheat oven to 300°F.

2. In a bowl, add the flaxseeds and chia, the olive oil and the sea salt to taste.

3. In a separate bowl, first whisk egg, and then add the egg white, the rosemary leaves and the water. Mix well.

4. Add the egg mixture to the flaxseed mixture and mix well until it becomes a homogeneous batter.

5. Let the dough rest for about one hour.

6. On a working surface lay down two pieces of parchment paper.

7. Put the dough on one of the papers and flatten roughly with a spoon.

8. Place the second paper on top and flatten the dough to about 1 inch thick.

9. Finely peel the paper off the top.

10. Cut the dough into squares and place in a baking sheet.

11. Bake for 30 minutes, then peel off the paper and flip over to cool.

Servings: 24

Cooking Time

Inactive Time: 1 hour

Total Time: 45 minutes

Nutrition Facts

Serving size: 1/24 of a recipe (0.7 ounces).

Percent daily values based on the Reference Daily Intake (RDI) for a 2000 calorie diet.

Amount Per Serving

Calories 24.1

Calories From Fat (52%) 12.5

% Daily Value

Total Fat 1.5g 2%

Saturated Fat 0.2g 1%

Cholesterol 7.8mg 3%

Sodium 6.2mg <1%

Potassium 11.9mg <1%

Total Carbohydrates 1.5g <1%

Fiber 1.6g 6%

Sugar 0.0g

Protein 1.1g 2%

Tuna Avocado Burgers

Ingredients

2 cans of tuna

2 Tbsp cream cheese

1 avocado

2 Tbsp grated cheddar cheese

3 Tbsp almond flour

salt, pepper, garlic powder

coconut oil

Instructions

1. Pour the drained tuna into a bowl.

2. Add in the cream cheese, cheddar cheese and spices and mix well. Add sliced avocado to the mixture.

3. Stir the mixture between your hands and make balls. Roll the balls in almond flour.

4. Heat your frying pan at moderate temperature to allow the coconut oil to melt.

5. Cook the tuna burgers three minutes per side (when done, the patties will be browned on the outside).

6. Serve hot.

Servings: 4

Cooking Time

Total Time: 20 minutes

Nutrition Facts

Serving size: 1/4 of a recipe (3.5 ounces)

Percent daily values based on the Reference Daily Intake (RDI) for a 2000 calorie diet.

Amount Per Serving

Calories 194.1

Calories From Fat (61%) 118.4

% Daily Value

Total Fat 13.9g 21%

Saturated Fat 3.1g 15%

Cholesterol 26.2mg 9%

Sodium 201.1mg 8%

Potassium 375.1mg 11%

Total Carbohydrates 5.3g 2%

Fiber 3.7g 15%

Sugar 0.6g

Protein 13.5g 27%

FAT BOMBS (SAVORY AND SWEET)

Cheesy Basil Sausage Fat Bombs

Ingredients

1 Italian sausage, chopped

2 Tbsp yogurt cream cheese, room temperature

2 Tbsp ricotta or cottage cheese

2 Tbsp unsalted butter

1 tsp garlic, minced

1/2 tsp fresh basil (chopped)

4 Tbsp pecan halves, toasted & chopped

parmesan cheese (grated)

Instructions

1. In a bowl, mix chopped sausage, cream cheese, ricotta cheese, butter, chopped basil, garlic and pecans.

2. Make 4 balls, place them on a plate and sprinkle with parmesan cheese.

3. Refrigerate for 4 hours.

4. Serve.

Servings: 4

Cooking Time

Total Time: 10 minutes

Nutrition Facts

Serving size: 1/4 of a recipe (2.1 ounces)

Percent daily values based on the Reference Daily Intake (RDI) for a 2000 calorie diet.

Amount Per Serving

Calories 202.9

Calories From Fat (82%) 167.3

% Daily Value

Total Fat 19.2g 30%

Saturated Fat 7.4g 37%

Cholesterol 47.1mg 16%

Sodium 193.8mg 8%

Potassium 60.9mg 2%

Total Carbohydrates 2.4g <1%

Fiber 0.8g 3%

Sugar 0.5g

Protein 6.6g 13%

Choco-Coco Peppermint Fat Bombs

Ingredients

3 cup melted coconut butter

1 cup finely shredded, unsweetened coconut

3 Tbsp coconut oil, melted

1 tsp pure peppermint extract

2 Tbsp cacao powder

Instructions

1. Mix together melted coconut butter, shredded coconut, 1 tablespoon of coconut oil and peppermint extract.

2. Pour coconut butter mixture into mini muffin tins that have been lined with paper liners. Fill halfway.

3. Place in refrigerator and allow to harden for about 15 minutes.

4. In a bowl, mix together 2 tablespoons coconut oil and cacao powder.

5. Remove muffin tin from refrigerator and top each muffin with chocolate mixture.

6. Return to refrigerator until the chocolate has set.

7. Serve.

Servings: 8

Nutrition Facts

Serving size: 1/8 of a recipe (1.6 ounces)

Percent daily values based on the Reference Daily Intake (RDI) for a 2000 calorie diet.

Amount Per Serving

Calories 124.2

Calories From Fat (97%) 120.2

% Daily Value

Total Fat 13.6g 21%

Saturated Fat 11.0g 55%

Cholesterol 0mg 0%

Sodium 89.6mg 4%

Potassium 33.5mg <1%

Total Carbohydrates 1.3g <1%

Fiber 0.7g 3%

Sugar 0.2g

Protein 0.4g <1%

Coconut Fat Bombs

Ingredients

1/3 cup coconut oil, melted

1 Tbsp shredded coconut

1/3 cup coconut butter, softened

1 tsp granulated sweetener of choice, to taste

Instructions

1. Prepare ice cube trays.

2. Mix all the ingredients in a deep bowl until your natural sweetener is completely dissolved.

3. Pour batter into ice cube trays.

4. Place in refrigerator for two minutes.

5. Serve and enjoy!

Servings: 8

Cooking Time

Total Time: 5 minutes

Nutrition Facts

Serving size: 1/8 of a recipe (1.3 ounces)

Percent daily values based on the Reference Daily Intake (RDI) for a 2000 calorie diet.

Amount Per Serving

Calories 161.2

Calories From Fat (92%) 148.7

% Daily Value

Total Fat 16.9g 26%

Saturated Fat 13.5g 68%

Cholesterol 20.3mg 7%

Sodium 21.2mg <1%

Potassium 5.8mg <1%

Total Carbohydrates 3.0g <1%

Fiber 0.1g <1%

Sugar 0.3g

Protein 0.2g <1%

Macadamia Fat Bombs

Ingredients

3 Tbsp macadamia nuts

5 Tbsp cocoa powder, unsweetened

½ cup coconut oil

2 Tbsp granulated stevia (or sweetener to your choice)

coarse sea salt, to taste

Instructions

1. Melt the coconut oil in a saucepan. Add cocoa powder and the sweetener of your choice.

2. Mix and remove from heat. Add in the chopped nuts and mix well.

3. Pour cocoa and nuts mixture into silicone molds about 3/4 full.

4. Refrigerate for several hours until completely hardened.

5. Before serving, remove from silicone molds and place on a serving dish.

6. Serve and enjoy!

Servings: 8

Cooking Time

Total Time: 20 minutes

Nutrition Facts

Serving size: 1/8 of a recipe (1 ounces)

Percent daily values based on the Reference Daily Intake (RDI) for a 2000 calorie diet.

Amount Per Serving

Calories 201.5

Calories From Fat (94%) 188.8

% Daily Value

Total Fat 22.1g 34%

Saturated Fat 13.3g 67%

Cholesterol 0mg 0%

Sodium 1.2mg <1%

Potassium 90.6mg 3%

Total Carbohydrates 3.4g 1%

Fiber 2.0g 8%

Sugar 0.5g

Protein 1.5g 3%

Nutmeg and Cinnamon Fat Bombs

Ingredients

½ cup butter

1/3 cup shredded coconut, unsweetened

1 pinch ground nutmeg

2 pinches ground cinnamon

1 tsp vanilla extract

Instructions

1. Place the butter in a bowl and let melt to room temperature.

2. In a separate bowl, mix together butter, half of the shredded coconut, nutmeg and cinnamon.

3. Make several small-sized balls. Roll in the shredded coconut.

4. Store in refrigerator or freezer for several hours.

Servings: 6

Cooking Time

Total Time: 10 minutes

Nutrition Facts

Serving size: 1/6 of a recipe (0.9 ounces)

Percent daily values based on the Reference Daily Intake (RDI) for a 2000 calorie diet.

Amount Per Serving

Calories 136.6

Calories From Fat (99%) 135.1

% Daily Value

Total Fat 15.4g 24%

Saturated Fat 9.7g 49%

Cholesterol 40.7mg 14%

Sodium 2.1mg <1%

Potassium 5.4mg <1%

Total Carbohydrates 0.1g <1%

Fiber 0.1g <1%

Sugar 0.1g

Protein 0.2g <1%

Rich Bacon Fat Bombs

Ingredients

½ cup butter

4 strips bacon, sliced into small strips

1 ½ green onion, finely diced

2 tsp Worcestershire for steaks

½ tsp black pepper

2 slices bacon, crumbled

Instructions

1. Melt 1 tablespoon butter in a frying pan on medium heat and add in bacon pieces.

2. Add in finely diced onion and fry until onion and bacon are crispy.

3. Set aside and cool to room temp.

4. Add softened butter to a large mixing bowl.

5. Add in bacon and onions, Worcestershire for steaks, and pepper.

6. Use the electric mixer and cream together all ingredients. Roll in the crumbled bacon.

7. Place in refrigerator for 4 hours.

Servings: 6

Cooking Time

Total Time: 15 minutes

Nutrition Facts

Serving size: 1/6 of a recipe (3.2 ounces)

Percent daily values based on the Reference Daily Intake (RDI) for a 2000 calorie diet.

Amount Per Serving

Calories 323.6

Calories From Fat (89%) 289.5

% Daily Value

Total Fat 32.5g 50%

Saturated Fat 15.4g 77%

Cholesterol 66.5mg 22%

Sodium 336.2mg 14%

Potassium 143.9mg 4%

Total Carbohydrates 3.6g 1%

Fiber 0.6g 2%

Sugar 1.5g

Protein 4.9g 10%

Savory Eggs and Lemongrass Fat Bombs

Ingredients

3 cups coconut oil

2 Tbsp organic butter

4 Tbsp cream cheese

3 slices crumbled bacon

4 whole eggs (boiled)

4 egg yolks (boiled)

1 stalk lemongrass

1 tsp freshly grated ginger

1 tsp fresh cilantro, chopped

zest of 1 lime

½ tsp fresh cilantro

1 tsp salt

Instructions

1. Place eggs in a pot and cover with water; for hardboiled eggs, you will need 10-12 minutes.

2. When done, let cool several minutes. Peel the eggs.

3. In a blender, place the coconut oil, organic butter, cream cheese, eggs, yolks, bacon, lemongrass, ginger, lime zest, cilantro and salt. Blend until smooth.

4. Make balls and place in a freezer overnight.

5. Serve.

Servings: 8

Cooking Time

Total Time: 20 minutes

Nutrition Facts

Serving size: 1/8 of a recipe (3.1 ounces)

Percent daily values based on the Reference Daily Intake (RDI) for a 2000 calorie diet.

Amount Per Serving

Calories 342.0

Calories From Fat (91%) 311.6

% Daily Value

Total Fat 35.6g 55%

Saturated Fat 23.9g 120%

Cholesterol 204.4mg 68%

Sodium 315.7mg 13%

Potassium 81.1mg 2%

Total Carbohydrates 0.8g <1%

Fiber 0.0g <1%

Sugar 0.3g

Protein 6.4g 13%

Speedy Pepperoni Fat Bombs

Ingredients

4 slices pepperoni sausages

3 slices pancetta bacon

1/2 cup yogurt cream cheese

1 chili pepper (or jalapeno)

hot paprika (or smoked paprika)

1/2 tsp dried basil

1/4 tsp onion powder

1/4 tsp garlic powder

salt and pepper to taste

Instructions

1. In a bowl, mix all ingredients – chopped pepperoni sausages, pancetta bacon, cream cheese, pepper, spices – and add salt to taste.

2. Mix with the spoon to get a compact mixture.

3. Make 6 balls and refrigerate for 4 hours.

4. Serve.

Servings: 6

Cooking Time

Total Time: 15 minutes

Nutrition Facts

Serving size: 1/6 of a recipe (3.1 ounces)

Percent daily values based on the Reference Daily Intake (RDI) for a 2000 calorie diet.

Amount Per Serving

Calories 150.8

Calories From Fat (77%) 116.2

% Daily Value

Total Fat 13.2g 20%

Saturated Fat 5.5g 28%

Cholesterol 47.8mg 16%

Sodium 361.5mg 15%

Potassium 53.6mg 2%

Total Carbohydrates 2.5g <1%

Fiber 0.4g 2%

Sugar 0.6g

Protein 6.4g 13%

Victory Fat Bombs

Ingredients

½ cup cream cheese

¼ cup ghee

3 Tbsp mayonnaise

4 Tbsp crumbled bacon

1 Tbsp fresh herbs, finely chopped

salt and pepper to taste

grated cheese

Instructions

1. In a food processor mix cream cheese, ghee, mayonnaise and fresh herbs.

2. Place the cheese mass in a bowl and add in the crumbled bacon.

3. Stir lightly with the spoon. Roll in grated cheese.

4. With your hands create 6 balls and refrigerate them for 3 hours.

Servings: 6

Cooking Time

Total Time: 10 minutes

Nutrition Facts

Serving size: 1/6 of a recipe (2.3 ounces)

Percent daily values based on the Reference Daily Intake (RDI) for a 2000 calorie diet.

Amount Per Serving

Calories 210.8

Calories From Fat (87%) 182.7

% Daily Value

Total Fat 20.5g 32%

Saturated Fat 7.9g 39%

Cholesterol 40.4mg 13%

Sodium 325.4mg 14%

Potassium 80.0mg 2%

Total Carbohydrates 2.7g <1%

Fiber 0g 0%

Sugar 1.1g

Protein 4.2g 8%

Wacky Eggs Fat Bombs

Ingredients

6 fresh eggs

4 slices crumbled bacon

2 Tbsp coconut oil

1 Tbsp butter

2 oz cream cheese, softened

1/4 cup shredded Monterey Jack cheese

spices: garlic powder, onion powder, ground pepper, salt, parsley, basil, etc.

coconut flakes, unsweetened

Instructions

1. In small bowl, set aside the butter and oil together to melt at room temperature.

2. Whisk the eggs in a deep bowl. Add spices of your preference.

3. Heat the butter in a non-stick skillet over medium heat. Cook the eggs just for a while, switching off burner before completely done.

4. Put scrambled, slightly cooked eggs into another large bowl. Put in your cheeses and mix. Add bacon and stir.

5. Add the melted butter and coconut oil. Stir thoroughly.

6. Make into balls and roll into coconut flakes.

7. Freeze for about 30 minutes, or refrigerate for 4-5 hours.

Servings: 8

Cooking Time

Total Time: 10 minutes

Nutrition Facts

Serving size: 1/8 of a recipe (2.2 ounces)

Percent daily values based on the Reference Daily Intake (RDI) for a 2000 calorie diet.

Amount Per Serving

Calories 207.2

Calories From Fat (84%) 174.2

% Daily Value

Total Fat 19.6g 30%

Saturated Fat 9.6g 48%

Cholesterol 133.7mg 45%

Sodium 240.6mg 10%

Potassium 91.9mg 3%

Total Carbohydrates 0.6g <1%

Fiber 0g 0%

Sugar 0.4g

Protein 7.1g 14%

KETO SWEETS

Buckwheat Muffins with Nuts

Ingredients

2 ½ cups buckwheat flour

1 ½ cups walnuts, chopped

½ cup sweetener of your choice

4 Tbsp extra virgin olive oil

1 tsp pure vanilla extract

2 tsp baking powder

1 tsp baking soda

Instructions

1. Preheat oven to 345°F.

2. In a small bowl, whisk olive oil, sweetener of your choice and vanilla.

3. In a separate bowl, combine buckwheat flour, baking powder and baking soda. Add in chopped walnuts and toss to coat.

4. Add olive oil mixture to the flour mixture and stir slightly.

5. Spoon the batter into 12 muffin cups, filling 3/4 full.

6. Bake about 20 minutes. Allow to cool and serve.

Servings: 12

Cooking Time

Total Time: 30 minutes

Nutrition Facts

Serving size: 1/12 of a recipe (1.9 ounces)

Percent daily values based on the Reference Daily Intake (RDI) for a 2000 calorie diet.

Amount Per Serving

Calories 270.4

Calories From Fat (52%) 139.8

% Daily Value

Total Fat 16.5g 25%

Saturated Fat 1.6g 8%

Cholesterol 0mg 0%

Sodium 187.1mg 8%

Potassium 204.7mg 6%

Total Carbohydrates 14.2g 6%

Fiber 4.4g 18%

Sugar 1.7g

Protein 7.8g 16%

Keto Flaxseed Pancakes

Ingredients

½ cup ground flax seed meal

2 eggs

2 Tbsp butter, melted

¼ cup heavy cream

3 Tbsp cottage cheese

¼ tsp baking powder

olive oil for frying

Instructions

1. In a deep bowl, mix all ingredients together.

2. Heat the oil in a frying pan. Fry pancakes 2 minutes, flipping when bubbles appear in the middle and the edges turn slightly dry.

3. Cook one minute more on the other side.

4. Serve hot with your favorite cheese and enjoy!

Servings: 6

Nutrition Facts

Serving size: 1/6 of a recipe (1.8 ounces)

Percent daily values based on the Reference Daily Intake (RDI) for a 2000 calorie diet.

Amount Per Serving

Calories 154.8

Calories From Fat (73%) 112.5

% Daily Value

Total Fat 13.0g 20%

Saturated Fat 4.7g 23%

Cholesterol 80.3mg 27%

Sodium 91.5mg 4%

Potassium 143.4mg 4%

Total Carbohydrates 4.5g 2%

Fiber 3.5g 14%

Sugar 0.7g

Protein 6.1g 12%

Mirky Choco Truffles

Ingredients

3 cups almond flour

1 Tbsp flaxseed meal

1 Tbsp cocoa butter

5 Tbsp butter

1 Tbsp coconut oil

1 Tbsp sweetener of your choice

2 tsp vanilla extract

1 cup dark chocolate chips

chopped almonds

pinch of salt

Instructions

1. Combine butter, coconut oil, sweetener, vanilla, almond flour, flaxseed meal and salt in a large bowl.

2. With your hands knead the mixture until all ingredients are incorporated well.

3. Make balls and place them on a sheet of parchment paper; refrigerate for one hour.

4. In a double boiler, melt dark chocolate chips with the cocoa butter.

5. Dip each truffle in the melted chocolate, and place them back on the pan with parchment paper.

6. Refrigerate until the chocolate is completely firm. Serve!

Servings: 14

Cooking Time

Total Time: 50 minutes

Nutrition Facts

Serving size: 1/14 of a recipe (0.9 ounces)

Percent daily values based on the Reference Daily Intake (RDI) for a 2000 calorie diet.

Amount Per Serving

Calories 112.6

Calories From Fat (74%) 82.8

% Daily Value

Total Fat 9.9g 15%

Saturated Fat 2.5g 13%

Cholesterol 0mg 0%

Sodium 19.7mg <1%

Potassium 88.2mg 3%

Total Carbohydrates 5.0g 2%

Fiber 1.3g 5%

Sugar 1.1g

Protein 2.7g 5%

Peanut Butter Ice Cream

Ingredients

½ cup peanut butter, unsweetened

2 ½ cups whipped cream

9 oz cream cheese

1 tsp organic vanilla extract

½ cup sweetener of your choice

peanuts

Instructions

1. Mix all ingredients with an electric mixer until combined well. Adjust sweetener.

2. Pour mixture into a container and freeze for 2 hours.

3. Transfer ice cream mixture into a bowl and beat well with an electric mixer to avoid ice cream crystallization.

4. Freeze again for several hours.

5. Top with peanuts if desired.

6. Serve and enjoy!

Servings: 6

Cooking Time

Preparation Time: 15 minutes

Nutrition Facts

Serving size: 1/6 of a recipe (3.7 ounces)

Percent daily values based on the Reference Daily Intake (RDI) for a 2000 calorie diet.

Amount Per Serving

Calories 389.2

Calories From Fat (69%) 267.4

% Daily Value

Total Fat 31.0g 48%

Saturated Fat 13.9g 70%

Cholesterol 65.8mg 22%

Sodium 267.8mg 11%

Potassium 236.6mg 7%

Total Carbohydrates 21.6g 7%

Fiber 1.3g 5%

Sugar 16.7g

Protein 9.0g 18%

Three Ingredients Mango Cream

Ingredients

2 cups frozen mango

¾ cup heavy cream

10 drops sweetener of your choice

Instructions

1. Add the mango to a high speed blender and beat until it reaches a creamy consistency.

2. Add the heavy cream and continue to whip.

3. Freeze in container for 2 hours.

4. Serve.

Servings: 3

Cooking Time

Preparation Time: 10 minutes

Nutrition Facts

Serving size: 1/3 of a recipe (4.9 ounces)

Percent daily values based on the Reference Daily Intake (RDI) for a 2000 calorie diet.

Amount Per Serving

Calories 169.1

Calories From Fat (60%) 100.7

% Daily Value

Total Fat 11.5g 18%

Saturated Fat 7.0g 35%

Cholesterol 40.9mg 14%

Sodium 12.5mg <1%

Potassium 207.2mg 6%

Total Carbohydrates 12.3g 6%

Fiber 1.8g 7%

Sugar 7.1g

Protein 1.5g 3%

Total Minty Ice Cream

Ingredients

2 cups whipping cream

1 cup almond milk

4 egg yolks

5 drops green food coloring

¼ cup fresh mint leaves, or more to taste

1 tsp mint extract

1 tsp stevia powder (or sweetener of your choice)

Instructions

1. Microwave whipping cream and almond milk in microwave-safe bowl for 2 minutes.

2. In another bowl, combine all other ingredients. Add to heated whipped cream and stir until combined well.

3. Heat the mixture in a saucepan until thickened (but be very careful not to overcook it).

4. Strain into a bowl and chill for 30 minutes. Beat well with an electric mixer. Chill overnight in the fridge.

5. Serve in chilled glasses and enjoy.

Servings: 8

Cooking Time

Preparation Time: 20 minutes

Nutrition Facts

Serving size: 1/8 of a recipe (1.5 ounces)

Percent daily values based on the Reference Daily Intake (RDI) for a 2000 calorie diet.

Amount Per Serving

Calories 138.6

Calories From Fat (88%) 121.8

% Daily Value

Total Fat 13.8g 21%

Saturated Fat 8.0g 40%

Cholesterol 131.3mg 44%

Sodium 16.7mg <1%

Potassium 42.9mg 1%

Total Carbohydrates 2.1g <1%

Fiber 0.2g <1%

Sugar 0.8g

Protein 2.1g 4%

ELECTRIC PRESSURE COOKER

50 Easy Recipes for Healthy Eating, Healthy Living & Weight Loss

Modern Kitchen

INTRODUCTION TO ELECTRIC PRESSURE COOKER

Electric pressure cookers have been slowly making their way into kitchens across the world for a while now. While they are different from crockpots – the slow cookers that follow a 'set it and forget it' method – electric pressure cookers offer the same ease of use and peace of mind. Essentially, electric pressure cookers rely on – you guessed it! – pressure to cook the food. The airtight lid on the cooker locks in the moisture and the flavor while the food heats up and cooks thoroughly. Despite the fact that they rely on pressure, these instruments are extremely safe, as they have a safety valve that ensures the lid will not blow off. What's great about electric pressure cookers is that you do not need to stand over them like you would a traditional pot or pan; you can simply load in all of the necessary ingredients, turn the cooker to the desired heat setting, and be on your way. The only times you will need to come back to it are to stir the food and to release the lid when your meal is done cooking.

Aluminum or Stainless Steel?

While shopping for an electric pressure cooker, you'll see some models made of aluminum and some stainless steel ones. Those made of aluminum are cheaper, lighter, and offer superb heating performance that is generally very uniform in nature. However, these cookers may stain with routine use. So if you're on a budget, go for aluminum; just understand that you may need to replace your cooker sooner.

Cookers made of stainless steel are a bit heavier and costlier than their aluminum counterparts. But they are more durable, and you can use them for many more years. If buying this type of cooker, opt for one featuring a layered base. This is because stainless steel is not a very efficient heat conductor.

Size

Electric Pressure cookers come in different sizes; some of the most popular sizes are four quart, six quart and eight quart, which refers to liquid capacity. The four quart is ideal for couples and people living alone, the six quart is great for smaller families (up to four members), and the eight quart is superb for bigger families. So make sure you buy one that is appropriate for your daily cooking needs.

Ok, onto the recipes...

Enjoy!

50 EASY RECIPES

Balsamic Collard Greens Stew

Ingredients

1 bunch fresh collard greens

½ cup chicken broth

2 Tbsp olive oil

2 Tbsp tomato puree

1 small onion, sliced thin

3 minced garlic cloves

3 tsp balsamic vinegar

½ tsp salt

1 tsp sugar

Instructions

1. Soak fresh collard greens in cold water for 1 hour to remove dirt.

2. Meanwhile, put the chicken broth, tomato puree, oil, garlic, onion, and vinegar into the bottom of your electric pressure cooker and then stir to combine the ingredients.

3. Remove the greens from the water.

4. Remove the thickest parts of the stems at the base of the greens. Chop the stems into small pieces.

5. Place the collard greens on top of one another and roll them into cigar-shaped bundles. Cut the greens into 1–2 inch wide pieces.

6. Toss the greens and stems with sugar and salt. Add to the pot and drizzle with oil.

7. Close and lock the lead, and cook for 20 minutes.

8. When ready, use the Natural Release Method: simply remove the cooker from the heat and let the pressure drop naturally. Allow 5 to 20 minutes for this process.

9. Serve.

Servings: 4

Total Cooking Time: 30 minutes

Nutrition Facts

Serving size: ¼ of a recipe (5.4 ounces)

Percent daily values based on the Reference Daily Intake (RDI) for a 2000 calorie diet.

Amount Per Serving

Calories 110

Calories From Fat (58%) 64.1

% Daily Value

Total Fat 7.3g 11%

Saturated Fat 1g 5%

Cholesterol 0mg 0%

Sodium 410mg 17%

Potassium 218mg 6%

Total Carbohydrates 9.8g 3%

Fiber 3.2g 13%

Sugar 3.6g

Protein 3g 6%

Beef Barley with Herbs Soup

Ingredients

1 ¼ lbs. ground beef

2 ½ cups water

½ cup barley

1 can (15 oz.) crushed tomatoes

3 large carrots

2 stalks celery

1 large potato

1 medium onion

1 clove garlic

½ tsp dried basil

½ tsp dried marjoram

½ tsp dried thyme

½ tsp dried rosemary

¼ tsp salt

Fresh ground black pepper to taste

Instructions

1. Brown the beef in pressure cooker; drain off.

2. Add the water, tomatoes, and barley. Close and lock lid of your electric pressure cooker and bring it up to full pressure.

3. Reduce the heat to stabilize and cook for a further 10 minutes.

4. Meanwhile, split the carrots in half lengthwise and into thick slices.

5. Peel and dice potato and onion; mince the garlic.

6. After 10 minutes, release pressure, and then add the vegetables, thyme, basil, rosemary, salt, marjoram, and pepper to taste.

7. Close pressure cooker and bring it up to full pressure.

8. Reduce heat till pressure is stabilized and cook for10 minutes longer.

9. Release the pressure by the Natural Release Method.

Servings: 8

Total Cooking Time: 35 minutes

Nutrition Facts

Serving size: 1/8 of a recipe (7.3 ounces)

Percent daily values based on the Reference Daily Intake (RDI) for a 2000 calorie diet.

Amount Per Serving

Calories 280.8

Calories From Fat (54%) 152

% Daily Value

Total Fat 16.5g 25%

Saturated Fat 6.6g 33%

Cholesterol 58.8mg 20%

Sodium 166.8mg 7%

Potassium 495.7mg 14%

Total Carbohydrates 16.8g 6%

Fiber 3.81g 15%

Sugar 3.8g

Protein 16g 32%

Button Mushroom and Beef Stew

Ingredients

1 ½ lbs. beef

12 button mushrooms

1 onion, chopped

4 carrots, cut into chunks

4 potatoes

2 tsp dried parsley

1 ¼ cup condensed mushroom soup

2 cups water

2 Tbsp canola oil

1 cup beef broth (optional)

Instructions

1. Heat oil in bottom of your electric pressure cooker and brown the meat. Stir the meat until browned on all sides.

2. Add the onions, mushrooms, carrots, potatoes, pepper, salt, mushroom soup, parsley, water and beef broth.

3. Lock the pressure cooker. Bring it to high pressure over high heat. Cook 15 minutes.

4. Use the Natural Release Method.

5. Serve.

Servings: 8

Cooking Time

Total Time: 25 minutes

Nutrition Facts

Serving size: 1/8 of a recipe (11.6 ounces)

Percent daily values based on the Reference Daily Intake (RDI) for a 2000 calorie diet.

Amount Per Serving

Calories 367.9

Calories From Fat (60%) 220.6

% Daily Value

Total Fat 24.6g 38%

Saturated Fat 7.9g 39%

Cholesterol 48.7mg 16%

Sodium 327.8mg 14%

Potassium 787.5mg 23%

Total Carbohydrates 24.7g 8%

Fiber 3.7g 15%

Sugar 4.4g

Protein 12.8g 26%

Whiskied Chicken and Rice Stew

Ingredients

1 lb. skinless boneless chicken breasts

2 ½ cups water

1 cup orange juice

1 cup whiskey

1 ½ cups rice

2 onions, chopped

2 green bell peppers

4 carrots

3 cups vinegar

1 tsp sesame oil

1 Tbsp butter

1 cup orange juice

1 tsp red pepper flakes

2 tsp ground ginger

1 Tbsp corn starch

Salt and pepper to taste

Instructions

1. Place onions, green bell peppers, carrots and chicken in your electric pressure cooker.

2. In a bowl, mix orange juice, brown sugar, whiskey, vinegar, ginger, red pepper flakes, and sesame oil together in a bowl.

3. Discharge whiskey mix over chicken.

4. Close and lock the lid and provide full pressure for 15 minutes over medium heat.

5. Select Natural Release Method. Carefully open the lid and add the rice and water.

6. Close the lid. Cook at high pressure for 3 minutes and allow 10 minutes for natural release. Release the remaining pressure, and then open the lid quickly.

7. Mix butter into rice; stir it well.

8. Serve hot.

Servings: 8

Total Cooking Time: 55 minutes

Nutrition Facts

Serving size: 1/8 of a recipe (10.2 ounces)

Percent daily values based on the Reference Daily Intake (RDI) for a 2000 calorie diet.

Amount Per Serving

Calories 133.6

Calories From Fat (17%) 22.7

% Daily Value

Total Fat 3g 4%

Saturated Fat 1.2g 6%

Cholesterol 9mg 3%

Sodium 38.6mg 2%

Potassium 381.6mg 11%

Total Carbohydrates 17.9g 8%

Fiber 2.6g 10%

Sugar 8g

Protein 4g 8%

Collard Greens with Olives Salad

Ingredients

2 bunches collard greens, trimmed

1 ½ cups water

½ cup olives (green or black), sliced

Salt to taste

Olive oil

Lime

Instructions

1. Place the collard green stems in your electric pressure cooker and pour water to just cover the stems.

2. Close and lock the lid of the pressure cooker. Turn the heat up to high; when the cooker reaches pressure, lower to the heat to the minimum. Cook for 5-7 minutes at high pressure.

3. When time is up, open the cooker by the Natural Release Method.

4. Pull out the leaves and stems with tongs and put them on a small serving plate.

5. Add chopped olives and stir lightly. Dress salad with salt and olive oil before serving.

6. Sprinkle some lime juice. Enjoy!

Servings: 2

Total Cooking Time: 10 minutes

Nutrition Facts

Serving size: ½ of a recipe (10.6 ounces)

Percent daily values based on the Reference Daily Intake (RDI) for a 2000 calorie diet.

Amount Per Serving

Calories 60.9

Calories From Fat (50%) 30.7

% Daily Value

Total Fat 3.6g 6%

Saturated Fat 0.5g 2%

Cholesterol 0mg 0%

Sodium 313.9mg 13%

Potassium 155.8mg 4%

Total Carbohydrates 7.2g 2%

Fiber 3.3g 13%

Sugar 2.8g

Protein 1.4g 3%

Mustard Greens, Sausages and Beans Soup

Ingredients

2 cups mustard greens, chopped

15 oz. turkey sausage, chopped

1 can (11 oz.) white beans

1 onion, chopped

2 potatoes, chopped

1 bay leaf

3 garlic cloves, minced

2 cups vegetable broth

5 cups water

Salt and pepper to taste

Instructions

1. Turn on the browning feature of your electric pressure cooker.

2. Put in the onions, garlic and potatoes and sauté for about two minutes.

3. Add the white beans, bay leaf, water and vegetable stock. Season with salt and pepper to taste.

4. Set the pressure cooker to cook for 35 minutes. Adjust the valves to airtight and shut the lid to lock it into position.

5. When ready, release all pressure and unlock the lid.

6. Add the chopped sausage and the chopped mustard green leaves.

7. Adjust salt and pepper and stir well.

8. Set the pressure cooker to cook for 5 minutes. Adjust the valves to airtight and shut the lid to lock it into position.

9. When ready, use the Natural Release Method.

10. Serve hot.

Servings: 8

Total Cooking Time: 45 minutes

Nutrition Facts

Serving size: 1/8 of a recipe (11.9 ounces)

Percent daily values based on the Reference Daily Intake (RDI) for a 2000 calorie diet.

Amount Per Serving

Calories 306

Calories From Fat (31%) 96.3

% Daily Value

Total Fat 10.9g 17%

Saturated Fat 3g 15%

Cholesterol 42.5mg 14%

Sodium 463mg 19%

Potassium 993mg 28%

Total Carbohydrates 26g 11%

Fiber 8g 32%

Sugar 1g

Protein 19g 38%

Comme Crème Brûlée

Ingredients

8 egg yolks

6 Tbsp superfine sugar

1/3 cup granulated sugar

2 cups heavy cream

1 ½ tsp vanilla

Pinch of salt

Instructions

1. Add water to your electric pressure cooker and place the trivet in the bottom.

2. In a bowl, whisk egg yolks, granulated sugar and a pinch of salt. Add cream and vanilla and whisk until blended.

3. Strain into a large measuring bowl with pour spout, or a pitcher.

4. Pour mixture in to six custard cups, cover with foil, and place on trivet in pressure cooking pot.

5. Lock the lid in place. Select high pressure and set the timer for 6 minutes.

6. When ready, turn off pressure cooker and use the Natural Release Method. Carefully remove lid.

7. When cool, refrigerate covered with plastic wrap for at least 5 hours.

Servings: 6

Total Cooking Time: 20 minutes

Nutrition Facts

Serving size: 1/6 of a recipe (4.6 ounces)

Percent daily values based on the Reference Daily Intake (RDI) for a 2000 calorie diet.

Amount Per Serving

Calories 455.2

Calories From Fat (60%) 274

% Daily Value

Total Fat 31g 48%

Saturated Fat 17g 85%

Cholesterol 442mg 147%

Sodium 39.1mg 2%

Potassium 84mg 2%

Total Carbohydrates 38g 13%

Fiber 0g 0%

Sugar 29g

Protein 6.5g 13%

Beef with Cabbage and Potatoes

Ingredients

3 lbs. corned beef brisket

1 cabbage, cut into wedges

6 red potatoes, quartered

3 carrots

4 cups beef broth

1 large onion, quartered

8 cloves garlic

Instructions

1. Place the beef, onion, beef broth and garlic into the pressure cooking pot. Put a stand in the pressure cooking pot. Season with salt and pepper to taste.

2. Lock the lid in place. Choose high pressure and set the timer for 90 minutes.

3. After hearing the beep, turn off the pressure cooker.

4. Select Natural Release Method. When valve drops carefully remove the lid. Remove the stand and brisket from the pressure cooking pot.

5. Wrap the corned beef with aluminum foil until ready to serve.

6. Add the potatoes, carrots and cabbage to the broth in your electric pressure cooker. Lock the lid in place again.

7. Select high pressure and set the timer for 3 minutes.

8. After hearing the beep, turn off the pressure cooker do a quick pressure release.

9. After the valve drops carefully remove lid.

10. Serve hot.

Servings: 8

Total Cooking Time: 1 hour and 55 minutes

Nutrition Facts

Serving size: 1/8 of a recipe (15.6 ounces)

Percent daily values based on the Reference Daily Intake (RDI) for a 2000 calorie diet.

Amount Per Serving

Calories 443.2

Calories From Fat (53%) 233.2

% Daily Value

Total Fat 25.8g 40%

Saturated Fat 8.2g 41%

Cholesterol 91.8mg 31%

Sodium 1546mg 51%

Potassium 1217.5mg 35%

Total Carbohydrates 22.7g 8%

Fiber 2.91g 12%

Sugar 2.47g

Protein 29g 58%

Creamy Corn Soup

Ingredients

2 Tbsp unsalted butter

1 ½ cups leeks, chopped

6 ears of corn, kernels

2 cloves garlic, thinly sliced

2 bay leaves

¼ tsp fennel seed

3/4 quart low-sodium chicken stock

Kosher salt and freshly ground black pepper to taste

Extra-virgin olive oil, for serving

Croutons

Instructions

1. Melt butter over medium heat in your electric pressure cooker.

2. Add leeks and garlic and cook about 4 minutes, stirring frequently.

3. Add corn with cobs, fennel seed, bay leaves and enough chicken stock to barely cover corn; stir to combine.

4. Seal pressure cooker and bring to high pressure. Cook for 15 minutes.

5. Carefully release pressure using quick-release method and uncover.

6. Discard corn cobs and bay leaves.

7. Transfer the mixture to the blender (in batches); remove the central lid and cover the space with a folded kitchen towel.

8. Start blender slowly and gradually increase speed to high. Blend until completely smooth, adding more chicken stock or water as necessary.

9. Season with salt and pepper to taste.

10. Serve with croutons and a splash of oil.

Servings: 6

Cooking Time

Preparation Time: 25 minutes

Nutrition Facts

Serving size: 1/6 of a recipe (9.1 ounces).

Percent daily values based on the Reference Daily Intake (RDI) for a 2000 calorie diet.

Amount Per Serving

Calories 188.8

Calories From Fat (29%) 54.7

% Daily Value

Total Fat 6.2g 10%

Saturated Fat 3g 15%

Cholesterol 13.8mg 5%

Sodium 180mg 8%

Potassium 402.4mg 11%

Total Carbohydrates 30.58g 10%

Fiber 3.1g 12%

Sugar 2.8g

Protein 6.8g 14%

Creamy Swiss Chard Soup

Ingredients

1 ½ Tbsp unsalted butter

4 cups water

½ cup onion, chopped

4 cloves garlic

9 oz. potatoes

1 lb. Swiss chard

1 tsp dried vegetables mixture (any)

Salt and black ground pepper to taste

½ cup heavy cream

½ cup grated cheese, grated

Instructions

1. Melt butter in the pressure cooker and cook the onion and garlic; cover with water.

2. Bring to a boil, and then add the sliced potatoes, chopped Swiss chard and dried vegetables.

3. Close and lock the lid and cook for 10 minutes.

4. Select Natural Release Method.

5. Transfer the soup to a blender and process, adding heavy cream until soup is creamy and smooth. Adjust salt and pepper to taste.

6. Serve warm with grated cheese.

Servings: 6

Cooking Time

Total Time: 30 minutes

Nutrition Facts

Serving size: 1/6 of a recipe (11.7 ounces)

Percent daily values based on the Reference Daily Intake (RDI) for a 2000 calorie diet.

Amount Per Serving

Calories 164

Calories From Fat (58%) 95.7

% Daily Value

Total Fat 10.9g 17%

Saturated Fat 6.6g 33%

Cholesterol 36.7mg 12%

Sodium 239.8mg 10%

Potassium 515.8mg 15%

Total Carbohydrates 13g 4%

Fiber 2.4g 9%

Sugar 2.5g

Protein 5.1g 10%

Delectable Choco-Cheese

Ingredients

1 oz. chocolate, semisweet

1 ½ Tbsp cocoa powder, unsweetened

½ cup chocolate cookie crumbs

15 oz. cream cheese, softened

1 cup heavy whipping cream

1 Tbsp butter

1 tsp pure vanilla extract

2/3 cup brown sugar

1 pinch ground cinnamon

2 eggs

1 ½ cups water

Instructions

1. Place greased springform pan in your electric pressure cooker.

2. Mix the chocolate crumbs and cinnamon together. Place the crumb mixture on the bottom of the springform pan, pressing gently to form the crust.

3. In a bowl, mix butter and melted chocolate. Set aside.

4. In separate bowl, whisk cream cheese until smooth. Add chocolate mixture and process until well-mixed and combined.

5. Pour in the cream, vanilla extract, sugar, and eggs. Beat well.

6. Sift cocoa powder over batter and beat well until cocoa is totally incorporated.

7. Pour mixture over crumbs in pan. Cover cake with a piece of waxed paper. Wrap the entire pan with aluminum foil.

8. Add water to your electric pressure cooker. Place pan on the trivet in the pressure cooker.

9. Seal the cooker and bring it up to high pressure.

10. Reduce the heat to maintain the pressure and cook 45 to 50 minutes.

11. Remove cooker from heat and let the pressure drop by the Natural Release Method.

12. Remove cake from cooker and let cool to room temperature in pan.

13. Refrigerate chocolate cake for 8 hours before serving.

14. Serve and enjoy!

Servings: 10

Cooking Time

Total Time: 1 hour and 15 minutes

Nutrition Facts

Serving size: 1/10 of a recipe (4.8 ounces)

Percent daily values based on the Reference Daily Intake (RDI) for a 2000 calorie diet.

Amount Per Serving

Calories 342

Calories From Fat (69%) 235.5

% Daily Value

Total Fat 26.8g 41%

Saturated Fat 15.3g 76%

Cholesterol 119.7mg 40%

Sodium 204mg 9%

Potassium 135.4mg 4%

Total Carbohydrates 22.3g 7%

Fiber 0.6g 2%

Sugar 17.4g

Protein 4.9g 10%

Deuce Green Chili with Cilantro

Ingredients

3 lbs. bone-in skin-on chicken thighs

4 tomatoes, under-ripe

3 poblano peppers, chopped

2 chili peppers

2 jalapeño chilies, roughly chopped

1 white onion, roughly chopped

6 cloves garlic, peeled

1 Tbsp whole cumin seed, toasted and ground

Kosher salt to taste

1 Tbsp fresh lemon juice

½ cup fresh cilantro leaves, chopped

Instructions

1. Combine all ingredients except cilantro leaves in your electric pressure cooker.

2. Heat over high heat, then seal pressure cooker, bring to high pressure, and cook for 15 minutes.

3. Release pressure with Natural Release Method and carefully open the lid.

4. Transfer chicken pieces to a bowl and set aside.

5. Add cilantro to remaining contents of pressure cooker in a blender, or blend with a hand blender. Adjust salt to taste.

6. Return chicken to sauce, discarding skin and bones and shredding if desired.

7. Transfer chicken to a serving platter, garnish with chopped cilantro, and serve.

Servings: 6

Cooking Time

Total Time: 30 minutes

Nutrition Facts

Serving size: 1/6 of a recipe (15.5 ounces)

Percent daily values based on the Reference Daily Intake (RDI) for a 2000 calorie diet.

Amount Per Serving

Calories 360.1

Calories From Fat (29%) 103

% Daily Value

Total Fat 11.4g 18%

Saturated Fat 2.8g 14%

Cholesterol 208.3mg 69%

Sodium 509.9mg 21%

Potassium 992.3mg 28%

Total Carbohydrates 11.3g 4%

Fiber 3g 12%

Sugar 4.7g

Protein 26.4g 51%

Easy BBQ Pork

Ingredients

7 lbs. pork butt roast

2 11-oz. cans barbecue sauce

1 tsp garlic powder

Salt and pepper to taste

Instructions

1. Season the pork with garlic powder and salt and pepper to taste.

2. Place the pork in your electric pressure cooker.

3. Fill with water and close the lid; bring up to 15 pounds to pressure. Cook about 1 hour.

4. Release the pressure and drain off juices, reserving about two cups.

5. Shred the pork and mix with barbeque sauce, adding reserved liquid if needed.

6. Serve hot.

Servings: 6

Total Cooking Time: 1 hour and 10 minutes

Nutrition Facts

Serving size: 1/6 of a recipe (4.1 ounces)

Percent daily values based on the Reference Daily Intake (RDI) for a 2000 calorie diet.

Amount Per Serving

Calories 101.2

Calories From Fat (50%) 51

% Daily Value

Total Fat 5.7g 9%

Saturated Fat 2g 10%

Cholesterol 31mg 10%

Sodium 162.7mg 7%

Potassium 220mg 6%

Total Carbohydrates 4g 1%

Fiber 0.2g <1%

Sugar 3.2g

Protein 8.8g 18%

Easy and Quick Beef Pot Roast

Ingredients

3 pound boneless beef chuck roast

4 carrots

4 potatoes

1 can (14.5 oz.) beef broth

1 ½ Tbsp Worcestershire sauce

1 large onion, cut into 4 wedges

2 Tbsp vegetable oil

Salt and ground black pepper to taste

1 pinch onion powder

Instructions

1. Heat oil in your electric pressure cooker over medium-high heat.

2. Brown the roast on all sides within the hot oil; season with pepper and onion powder.

3. Pour in beef broth and sauce, add chopped onion, and lock the lid.

4. Bring the pressure cooker up to full pressure and cook for half an hour.

5. Use the Natural Release Method to release the pressure.

6. Add the carrots and potatoes, mix, and seal the lid once more.

7. Cook on full pressure for 15 minutes.

8. Use the Natural Release Method once more and transfer the roast meat and vegetables to a dish.

9. Serve hot.

Servings: 6

Total Cooking Time: 1 hour and 10 minutes

Nutrition Facts

Serving size: 1/6 of a recipe (12.2 ounces)

Percent daily values based on the Reference Daily Intake (RDI) for a 2000 calorie diet.

Amount Per Serving

Calories 348

Calories From Fat (50%) 172.3

% Daily Value

Total Fat 19.2g 30%

Saturated Fat 6.4g 32%

Cholesterol 42.4mg 14%

Sodium 524.8mg 22%

Potassium 897.8mg 26%

Total Carbohydrates 29.4g 10%

Fiber 4.6g 18%

Sugar 4.8g

Protein 14.8g 30%

Easy Sautéed Vegetables

Ingredients

1 ½ lbs. Brussels sprouts

4 medium beets

1 ½ lbs. carrots

8 large cloves garlic, unpeeled

3 Tbsp olive oil

1 Tbsp chopped fresh thyme

Salt and ground black pepper to taste

Instructions

1. To your electric pressure cooker, add chopped vegetables, oil, salt and black pepper to taste.

2. Select sauté and cook under high pressure for 15 minutes.

3. When ready, select Natural Release Method. Carefully open the lid.

4. Transfer all vegetables from the cooker to the serving plate, toss well and serve.

Servings: 6

Total Cooking Time: 15 minutes

Nutrition Facts

Serving size: 1/6 of a recipe (10.2 ounces)

Percent daily values based on the Reference Daily Intake (RDI) for a 2000 calorie diet.

Amount Per Serving

Calories 178.8

Calories From Fat (37%) 65.6

% Daily Value

Total Fat 7.4g 11%

Saturated Fat 1g 5%

Cholesterol 0mg 0%

Sodium 149.4mg 6%

Potassium 984.2mg 28%

Total Carbohydrates 26.3g 9%

Fiber 9g 36%

Sugar 11.6g

Protein 5.8g 12%

Express 20 Lentil Soup

Ingredients

2 cups lentils

3 cups vegetable broth

3 cups water

1 onion, chopped

2 carrots

2 bay leaves

2 sprigs fresh thyme

1 potato, peeled and diced

¼ cup grated parmesan cheese (optional)

1 Tbsp olive oil

Salt and fresh ground black pepper to taste

Instructions

1. Heat the oil with your electric pressure cooker set to medium heat.

2. Add onion and sauté until soft, about 2 minutes.

3. Add carrots and sauté for another minute. Then add bay leaves, thyme, water and broth, potato and lentils; stir well.

4. Lock the lid in place on the cooker and bring the mixture to a boil over high heat till high pressure is achieved.

5. Reduce heat to maintain pressure for 6 minutes.

6. Remove from the heat and release the pressure naturally.

7. Open the lid very carefully.

8. Remove the bay leaves and thyme stems, and adjust salt and pepper.

9. Serve hot.

Servings: 8

Total Cooking Time: 20 minutes

Nutrition Facts

Serving size: 1/8 of a recipe (10 ounces)

Percent daily values based on the Reference Daily Intake (RDI) for a 2000 calorie diet.

Amount Per Serving

Calories 310.4

Calories From Fat (17%) 52.8

% Daily Value

Total Fat 6g 9%

Saturated Fat 1.5g 8%

Cholesterol 4.6mg 2%

Sodium 1461mg 61%

Potassium 824.2mg 24%

Total Carbohydrates 49.1g 16%

Fiber 14.9g 59%

Sugar 2.6g

Protein 15.8g 32%

Holiday Turkey Breast

Ingredients

4 lbs. turkey breast

3 cups orange juice

1 can cranberry sauce

1 package onion soup mix

Instructions

1. Place the turkey breast, skin-side down, into your electric pressure cooker.

2. Mix the orange juice, cranberry sauce and onion soup mix. Season with salt and pepper to taste.

3. Coat the turkey evenly with the sauce.

4. Set the pressure cooker to cook for 30 minutes. Close and lock the lid.

5. Adjust the valve to airtight and press start.

6. When the cooking cycle is complete, let the pressure drop naturally by itself. It should take about 15 minutes.

7. Remove the turkey breast from the juices and place on the serving plate.

8. Pour the sauce over the turkey and serve.

Servings: 6

Total Cooking Time: 45 minutes

Nutrition Facts

Serving size: 1/6 of a recipe (10.5 ounces)

Percent daily values based on the Reference Daily Intake (RDI) for a 2000 calorie diet.

Amount Per Serving

Calories 296.4

Calories From Fat (3%) 7.8

% Daily Value

Total Fat 0.9g 1%

Saturated Fat 0.2g 1%

Cholesterol 45.9mg 15%

Sodium 586.3mg 24%

Potassium 535.7mg 15%

Total Carbohydrates 53g 18%

Fiber 1.6g 6%

Sugar 45.7g

Protein 19.7g 39%

Homemade Applesauce

Ingredients

10 apples, peeled, cored & sliced

¼ cup sugar (or sweetener of your choice)

¼ cup apple juice

1 tsp ground cinnamon

½ tsp vanilla powder

Instructions

1. Place the apple pieces, apple juice, sugar, vanilla powder and cinnamon in your electric pressure cooker and stir to combine. Select high pressure and set cook time for 4 minutes.

2. Use the Natural Release Method.

3. Carefully remove the lid.

4. Stir applesauce until you've achieved your desired consistency.

5. Pour into glass jars or cups.

Servings: 4

Total Cooking Time: 10 minutes

Nutrition Facts

Serving size: ¼ of a recipe (12.3 ounces)

Percent daily values based on the Reference Daily Intake (RDI) for a 2000 calorie diet.

Amount Per Serving

Calories 210.7

Calories From Fat (2%) 3.7

% Daily Value

Total Fat 0.4g <1%

Saturated Fat 0.07g <1%

Cholesterol 0mg 0%

Sodium 0.8mg <1%

Potassium 306.7mg 9%

Total Carbohydrates 45.6g 17%

Fiber 4.5g 18%

Sugar 46.3g

Protein 0.9g 2%

Italiano Potato, Rice, & Spinach Soup

Ingredients

6 leeks

10 oz. fresh spinach

3 crushed garlic cloves

3 potatoes (cut in large chunks)

2 carrots

1 cup rice

3 cups chicken stock

3 cups water

½ cup olive oil

1 cup celery (chopped)

1 cup parsley (chopped)

2 Tbsp fresh lemon juice

3 Tbsp tomato paste

1 cup parmesan cheese (grated)

1 bay leaf

Salt and ground pepper to taste

2 tsp dried basil

Instructions

1. Heat oil in your electric pressure cooker.

2. Add garlic, leeks, and carrots and sauté in hot oil for 2 minutes.

3. Add rice and potatoes, stir well and cook for 1 minute.

4. Add broth, water, celery, parsley, bay leaf, salt and pepper to taste, basil, tomato paste and lemon juice. Stir well.

5. Secure the lid. On high heat, develop the steam to very high pressure.

6. Reduce the heat to maintain pressure, using a heat diffuser to maintain heat over burner, and cook for 4 minutes.

7. Release pressure with the Natural Release Method.

8. Remove the lid. Stir the soup well.

9. Ladle soup into bowls.

10. Sprinkle cheese over soup. Serve.

Servings: 8

Total Cooking Time: 35 minutes

Nutrition Facts

Serving size: 1/8 of a recipe (13.7 ounces)

Percent daily values based on the Reference Daily Intake (RDI) for a 2000 calorie diet.

Amount Per Serving

Calories 272.9

Calories From Fat (30%) 82.2

% Daily Value

Total Fat 9.3g 14%

Saturated Fat 1.8g 9%

Cholesterol 2.7mg <1%

Sodium 1000.9mg 42%

Potassium 849.3mg 24%

Total Carbohydrates 39.7g 13%

Fiber 5.3g 21%

Sugar 7.4g

Protein 9.6g 19%

Pork Sausage and Pepper Hash

Ingredients

10 pork sausages

1 can (15 ounces) diced tomatoes

1 can (15 ounces) tomato sauce

4 green bell peppers

1 cup water

1 Tbsp fresh basil

3 Tbsp garlic powder

1 Tbsp Italian seasoning

Salt and pepper to taste

Instructions

1. Combine tomatoes, tomato sauce, basil, garlic powder, Italian seasoning and water in your electric pressure cooker.

2. Add sausages to the sauce. Lay the peppers on top of the sausages, but don't mix.

3. Lock lid in place and set for high pressure. Set timer for 25 minutes and press start.

4. When beep sounds, turn off the pressure cooker and use the Natural Release Method.

5. When valve drops carefully remove the lid.

6. Serve hot immediately.

Servings: 6

Total Time: 30 minutes

Nutrition Facts

Serving size: 1/6 of a recipe (14.6 ounces)

Percent daily values based on the Reference Daily Intake (RDI) for a 2000 calorie diet.

Amount Per Serving

Calories 367.2

Calories From Fat (60%) 220

% Daily Value

Total Fat 24.8g 38%

Saturated Fat 6.8g 34%

Cholesterol 99.6mg 33%

Sodium 1328mg 55%

Potassium 624mg 18%

Total Carbohydrates 17.8g 6%

Fiber 4.3g 17%

Sugar 7.3g

Protein 22.2g 44%

Lamb in Red Wine Stew

Ingredients

6 lamb shanks

2 tomatoes

4 tsp flour

2 ½ Tbsp cold water

3 Tbsp olive oil

1 chopped onion

3 sliced carrots

3 cups red wine

1 cup vegetable stock

2 cloves crushed garlic

1 Tbsp fresh oregano

1 Tbsp lemon rind

Salt and fresh ground black pepper to taste

Instructions

1. Peel and clean the tomatoes and cut them into quarters.

2. Toss the shanks in the flour.

3. Heat half of the oil in your electric pressure cooker (no lid) and brown the shanks. Remove and set aside.

4. Add the remaining oil and the onion, carrots and garlic; cook for 5 minutes, stirring occasionally.

6. Add the tomatoes, oregano, lemon rind, wine and stock. Keep it boiling while stirring well for a few minutes.

7. Transfer the lamb shanks back to the cooker and season with salt and pepper to taste. Pour some of the sauce and vegetables over the meat.

8. Close and lock the lid. Set cooker to high pressure and cook for 25 minutes.

9. Use the Natural Release Method.

10. Simmer gravy and add the flour paste in slowly to thicken.

11. Serve.

Servings: 6

Total Cooking Time: 40 minutes

Nutrition Facts

Serving size: 1/6 of a recipe (9.6 ounces)

Percent daily values based on the Reference Daily Intake (RDI) for a 2000 calorie diet.

Amount Per Serving

Calories 351.2

Calories From Fat (57%) 200.6

% Daily Value

Total Fat 22.4g 34%

Saturated Fat 7.6g 38%

Cholesterol 76.1mg 25%

Sodium 126.4mg 5%

Potassium 617mg 18%

Total Carbohydrates 9.3g 3%

Fiber 2.2g 9%

Sugar 4.2g

Protein 22.3g 45%

Lentils and Carrot Soup

Ingredients

2 cups brown lentils

3 cups vegetable broth

3 cups water

1 medium onion, chopped

2 large carrots, peeled and finely chopped

2 bay leaves

2 sprigs fresh thyme

1 medium potato, peeled and diced

1 tsp fresh winter savory (optional)

1 Tbsp olive oil

¼ cup grated parmesan cheese (optional)

Salt and fresh ground black pepper to taste

Instructions

1. Sauté the onion with oil in your electric pressure cooker about 2 minutes.

2. Add chopped carrots and sauté for another minute. Add bay leaves, savory, thyme, water, broth, potato and lentils. Stir well.

3. Close and lock the lid in place on the cooker and bring the mixture to a boil over high heat till high pressure is achieved.

4. Reduce heat to maintain pressure for 6 minutes.

5. Remove from the heat and use the Natural Release Method. Carefully open the lid, pointing it away from you.

6. Remove the bay leaves and thyme stems and adjust salt and pepper to taste.

8. Serve hot.

Servings: 8

Total Cooking Time: 20 minutes

Nutrition Facts

Serving size: 1/8 of a recipe (10.3 ounces)

Percent daily values based on the Reference Daily Intake (RDI) for a 2000 calorie diet.

Amount Per Serving

Calories 292

Calories From Fat (14%) 41.1

% Daily Value

Total Fat 4.6g 7%

Saturated Fat 1.2g 6%

Cholesterol 3.7mg 1%

Sodium 679.3mg 28%

Potassium 794.9mg 23%

Total Carbohydrates 42.1g 15%

Fiber 17.3g 69%

Sugar 2.8g

Protein 16.7g 33%

Mediterranean Chicken, Sausage and Lentil Soup

Ingredients

1 skinless, bone-in chicken breast half

4 Italian turkey sausage links

1 cup green lentils

1 cup chopped fresh parsley

2 tsp olive oil

1 (15 ounce) can garbanzo beans

1 diced medium onion

4 minced cloves garlic

1 cup pearl barley

3 cups chicken stock

1 cup mild salsa

Instructions

1. Heat the olive oil in your electric pressure cooker, add sausage, and cook until it appears browned. Remove sausage to a bowl and set aside.

2. Add additional olive oil to electric pressure cooker and then cook onion and garlic till onion is golden-

brown and transparent. Next, add garbanzo beans and mix 1 minute.

3. Place sausage in the pressure cooker. Add lentils, parsley, chicken, and chicken stock to cooker, adding water if necessary to fully cover chicken.

4. Close and lock lid and place pressure regulator on vent pipe.

5. Bring your pressure cooker to full pressure over high heat (it may take 15 minutes).

6. Decrease heat to medium high and cook for another 9 minutes.

7. Let the pressure drop naturally using the Natural Release Method.

8. Open cooker, remove chicken and shred meat, then return to soup.

9. Serve hot.

Servings: 8

Total Cooking Time: 50 minutes

Nutrition Facts

Serving size: 1/8 of a recipe (9.2 ounces)

Percent daily values based on the Reference Daily Intake (RDI) for a 2000 calorie diet.

Amount Per Serving

Calories 285.6

Calories From Fat (20%) 57.3

% Daily Value

Total Fat 6.4g 10%

Saturated Fat 2g 10%

Cholesterol 21.7mg 7%

Sodium 807.3mg 34%

Potassium 644.6mg 18%

Total Carbohydrates 32g 11%

Fiber 11.4g 46%

Sugar 2.5g

Protein 21.6g 43%

Minestrone Tortellini with Parmesan Cheese

Ingredients

8 oz. dry tortellini

4 cups vegetable broth

24 oz. spaghetti sauce

1 can diced tomatoes

2 Tbsp olive oil

1 white onion, diced

2 stalks celery, sliced

2 carrots, sliced

1 ½ tsp Italian seasoning

1 Tbsp fresh garlic, minced

1 tsp sugar

Salt and pepper to taste

Instructions

1. Add oil to the pressure cooker and heat on high with the lid off till it appears brown.

2. Sauté onions, carrots, celery, and garlic 3-4 minutes. Add the remaining ingredients and stir well.

3. Lock on the pressure cooker's lid, set the cooker to high and cook for 5 minutes.

4. Select Natural Release Method to let the pressure drop naturally.

5. Serve with shredded parmesan cheese.

Servings: 6

Total Cooking Time: 20 minutes

Nutrition Facts

Serving size: 1/6 of a recipe (13 ounces)

Percent daily values based on the Reference Daily Intake (RDI) for a 2000 calorie diet.

Amount Per Serving

Calories 318

Calories From Fat (31%) 98.2

% Daily Value

Total Fat 11g 17%

Saturated Fat 2.5g 12%

Cholesterol 28.7mg 10%

Sodium 1587mg 66%

Potassium 607.7mg 17%

Total Carbohydrates 44.5g 15%

Fiber 5.9g 23%

Sugar 6.6g

Protein 11.2g 22%

Pork Shoulder with Jalapeño Peppers

Ingredients

3 lbs. boneless pork shoulder

1 ½ cups beef broth

1 cup water

1 large onion, chopped

4 cloves garlic

2 fresh poblano peppers (roughly chopped)

3 jalapeño peppers (roughly chopped)

1 serrano pepper (roughly chopped)

2 tsp ground coriander

3 tsp ground cumin

3 Tbsp olive oil

Instructions

1. Add oil to your electric pressure cooker and brown the pork shoulder from all sides.

2. Add all ingredients from the list and cover with water and beef broth.

3. Close the lid and bring up to 15 pounds of pressure. Cook for 1 hour.

4. Select Natural Release Method and carefully open the lid.

5. Serve hot.

Servings: 8

Total Cooking Time: 1 hour and 10 minutes

Nutrition Facts

Serving size: 1/8 of a recipe (8.6 ounces)

Percent daily values based on the Reference Daily Intake (RDI) for a 2000 calorie diet.

Amount Per Serving

Calories 380.5

Calories From Fat (63%) 239.7

% Daily Value

Total Fat 26.7g 41%

Saturated Fat 7.9g 39%

Cholesterol 105.5mg 35%

Sodium 273.7mg 11%

Potassium 628.7mg 18%

Total Carbohydrates 2.9g <1%

Fiber 0.8g 3%

Sugar 0.9g

Protein 30.7g 61%

Pot Roast in Peach Juice

Ingredients

3 ½ lbs. beef roast

6 cups peach juice

2 Tbsp olive oil

2 onions, peeled & quartered

3 garlic cloves, smashed

3 ½ Tbsp cornstarch

3 oz. cold water

Salt and pepper to taste

Instructions

1. Heat the oil in the pressure cooker and brown the roast.

2. When the roast is browned attractively on both sides, add the garlic and onion.

3. Pour in enough peach juice to fully cover the roast.

4. Put on the pressure cooker lid. Start your timer when pressure begins to escape. 45 minutes is needed to make the meat fork-tender.

5. After 45 minutes, remove the pressure cooker from heat and allow it to rest about 15 minutes. Open the

valve. When all pressure is released, carefully remove the lid. Place your roast in a bowl and allow to rest.

6. Make a slurry of the corn starch with cold water. Bring the pot liquid to the boil, then stir the slurry once again and pour into the pot liquid until it thickens.

7. Pour sauce over the meat and serve.

Servings: 10

Total Cooking Time: 55 minutes

Nutrition Facts

Serving size: 1/10 of a recipe (11.4 ounces)

Percent daily values based on the Reference Daily Intake (RDI) for a 2000 calorie diet.

Amount Per Serving

Calories 476.7

Calories From Fat (60%) 284.7

% Daily Value

Total Fat 30.9g 48%

Saturated Fat 11.7g 59%

Cholesterol 102mg 34%

Sodium 102.9mg 4%

Potassium 564.5mg 16%

Total Carbohydrates 24g 8%

Fiber 1.9g 8%

Sugar 1g

Protein 25g 50%

Potato and Cheddar Cheese Soup

Ingredients

4 potatoes, peeled and cut

3 cups cheddar cheese, grated

4 small onions, chopped

1 ½ cups water

4 cups milk

1 Tbsp parsley, chopped

Salt and pepper to taste

Instructions

1. Put potatoes, onions, salt and water in your electric pressure cooker.

2. Close the lid and set at high heat for full pressure.

3. Reduce heat and cook for 3 minutes.

4. Select Natural Release Method and cool naturally till there is no pressure inside cooker.

5. Carefully open the pressure cooker.

6. Mix the contents smoothly in a blender or mash through a sieve.

7. Return soup to cooker and add milk and pepper.

8. Place the cooker on medium heat and bring to a boil, stirring continuously.

9. Add cheese and stir till cheese melts.

10. Serve hot.

Servings: 10

Total Cooking Time: 25 minutes

Nutrition Facts

Serving size: 1/10 of a recipe (9.3 ounces)

Percent daily values based on the Reference Daily Intake (RDI) for a 2000 calorie diet.

Amount Per Serving

Calories 284.8

Calories From Fat (47%) 133.8

% Daily Value

Total Fat 15.2g 23%

Saturated Fat 9.6g 48%

Cholesterol 49.4mg 16%

Sodium 763.5mg 32%

Potassium 558.9mg 16%

Total Carbohydrates 22.6g 8%

Fiber 2.5g 10%

Sugar 7.8g

Protein 15.1g 30%

Piquant Pork Chops

Ingredients

8 pork chops

1 cup water (or broth)

1 small onion

2 carrots

5 medium potatoes, diced

3 Tbsp Worcestershire sauce

¼ cup butter

Salt and black ground pepper to taste

Instructions

1. Place the pork chops with oil in your electric pressure cooker.

2. Add salt and pepper to taste and brown pork chops on both sides.

3. Clean and peel potatoes and carrots and add to the meat.

4. Cut the onion into small pieces and add to the cooker.

5. Pour in the water or broth.

6. Lock the lid and bring to high pressure; once pressure is established, set timer for 15 minutes.

7. Use the Natural Release Method to let the pressure drop naturally over 5 to 20 minutes.

8. Serve hot.

Servings: 8

Cooking Time

Total Time: 25 minutes

Nutrition Facts

Serving size: 1/8 of a recipe (8.6 ounces)

Percent daily values based on the Reference Daily Intake (RDI) for a 2000 calorie diet.

Amount Per Serving

Calories 250.9

Calories From Fat (32%) 80.2

% Daily Value

Total Fat 9g 14%

Saturated Fat 4.8g 24%

Cholesterol 76.6mg 26%

Sodium 115.8mg 5%

Potassium 822.5mg 24%

Total Carbohydrates 18.7g 6%

Fiber 2.3g 9%

Sugar 2g

Protein 22.9g 46%

Homemade Chicken Stock

Ingredients

2 ½ lbs. chicken thighs

2 chicken feet (optional)

2 carrots

1 onion, unpeeled, quartered

1 celery rib, cut into 1-inch pieces

4 whole peppercorns

8 cups water

Instructions

1. Combine all the ingredients in your electric pressure cooker.

2. Cover and lock the lid; bring up to high pressure.

3. Reduce the heat so that it can be jiggled about 2-4 times per minute and cook for a further 25 minutes.

4. Release the pressure over 5 to 20 minutes using the Natural Release Method.

5. Strain the stock and refrigerate till the fat hardens.

6. Remove the fat and keep refrigerated up to 3 days.

Servings: 8

Total Cooking Time: 50 minutes

Nutrition Facts

Serving size: 1/8 of a recipe (14.2 ounces)

Percent daily values based on the Reference Daily Intake (RDI) for a 2000 calorie diet.

Amount Per Serving

Calories 35.6

Calories From Fat (22%) 7.7

% Daily Value

Total Fat 0.8g 1%

Saturated Fat 0.2g 1%

Cholesterol 0mg 0%

Sodium 422.8mg 18%

Potassium 203.4mg 6%

Total Carbohydrates 3.9g 1%

Fiber 0.9g 3%

Sugar 2g

Protein 3g 6%

Red Potato Salad with Dill

Ingredients

6 medium red potatoes

3 hardboiled eggs, chopped

2 Tbsp chopped fresh dill

1 cup light mayonnaise

1 cup water

1 cup chopped onion

1 stalk fresh celery (chopped)

1 tsp yellow mustard

1 tsp apple cider vinegar

Salt and black ground pepper to taste

Instructions

1. Place potatoes in your electric pressure cooker and cover with water.

2. Close and lock the lid. Cook on high pressure for 3 minutes.

3. Let steam release for 3 minutes, then quickly release pressure and open cookware.

4. Peel and dice potatoes once they are cool enough to handle.

5. Make layers of potatoes, onion, and celery in large bowl.

6. Season every layer with salt and pepper to taste.

7. Top with the sliced eggs and sprinkle with dill.

8. In a separate bowl mix the mayonnaise, mustard, vinegar and toss.

9. Add the mayo mixture to the potatoes and stir lightly.

10. Chill 1 to 2 hours before serving.

Servings: 4

Total Cooking Time: 30 minutes

Nutrition Facts

Serving size: ¼ of a recipe (12 ounces)

Percent daily values based on the Reference Daily Intake (RDI) for a 2000 calorie diet.

Amount Per Serving

Calories 321.7

Calories From Fat (41%) 132.9

% Daily Value

Total Fat 14.7g 23%

Saturated Fat 2.9g 15%

Cholesterol 169.6mg 57%

Sodium 331.7mg 14%

Potassium 1161.4mg 33%

Total Carbohydrates 33.1g 13%

Fiber 3.6g 14%

Sugar 2.4g

Protein 9.9g 20%

Whole Chicken

Ingredients

2 lb. whole chicken

1 ½ cups chicken broth or water

2 Tbsp olive oil

Salt and black pepper to taste

Instructions

1. Rinse chicken and pat dry. Season with salt and pepper.

2. In uncovered pressure cooker, heat oil and brown the chicken on all sides.

3. Remove chicken. Place stand in pressure cooker and place browned chicken in the stand.

4. Add water or broth around chicken. Put the lid on cooker, seal, and bring up to pressure. Cook for 25 minutes.

5. Release pressure by Natural Release Method over 5 to 20 minutes.

6. Transfer chicken to serving plate and serve.

Servings: 4

Total Cooking Time: 30 minutes

Nutrition Facts

Serving size: ¼ of a recipe (5.8 ounces)

Percent daily values based on the Reference Daily Intake (RDI) for a 2000 calorie diet.

Amount Per Serving

Calories 84.8

Calories From Fat (80%) 68.2

% Daily Value

Total Fat 7.6g 12%

Saturated Fat 1.2g 6%

Cholesterol 0mg 0%

Sodium 481.4mg 20%

Potassium 135.3mg 4%

Total Carbohydrates 0.6g <1%

Fiber 0g 0%

Sugar 0.5g

Protein 3.2g 6%

Pumpkin Pie with Pecans

Ingredients

Crust

½ cup pecan cookies (or any other cookies)

1/3 cup toasted pecans, chopped

2 Tbsp butter, melted

Filling

1 ½ tsp pumpkin pie spice

1 egg, beaten

1 ½ cups pure solid-pack pumpkin

½ cup light brown sugar

½ cup evaporated milk

½ tsp salt

Instructions

1. In a bowl, mix chopped pecans, pecan cookie crumbs and butter.

2. Spread evenly in the bottom and about an inch up the side of a springform pan. Place in the freezer for 15 minutes.

3. Meanwhile combine in a large bowl the pumpkin pie spice, sugar and salt. Whisk in egg, evaporated milk and pumpkin.

4. Pour into pie crust. Cover top of springform pan with aluminum foil.

5. Pour 1 cup water into your electric pressure cooker and place the trivet in the bottom.

6. Carefully center the filled pan on a foil sling and lower it into the pressure cooking pot.

7. Lock the lid in place. Select high pressure and set the timer for 35 minutes.

8. When ready, use Natural Release Method. When valve drops, carefully remove lid.

9. Remove aluminum foil. When pie is cooled, refrigerate covered with plastic wrap for at least 4 hours.

Servings: 6

Cooking Time

Inactive Time: 4 hours

Total Time: 15 minutes

Nutrition Facts

Serving size: 1/6 of a recipe (4.3 ounces)

Percent daily values based on the Reference Daily Intake (RDI) for a 2000 calorie diet.

Amount Per Serving

Calories 217.8

Calories From Fat (45%) 97.5

% Daily Value

Total Fat 11.3g 17%

Saturated Fat 4.3g 21%

Cholesterol 47.9mg 16%

Sodium 387.7mg 16%

Potassium 256mg 7%

Total Carbohydrates 27.4g 9%

Fiber 2.4g 10%

Sugar 22.8g

Protein 3.9g 8%

Retro Beef with Mushrooms and Chestnuts

Ingredients

1 ½ lbs. beef meat

8 oz. mushrooms

8 oz. sliced water chestnuts

1 large onion, diced

3 cups celery, sliced

3 Tbsp soy sauce

2 Tbsp molasses

Bean sprouts, fresh

1 Tbsp shortening

Salt and ground pepper to taste

1 cup water

Flour

Instructions

1. Slice beef thinly.

2. Dust the meat lightly with seasoned flour. Add to your electric pressure cooker and brown in batches in hot, smoky oil.

3. Add celery, onion, soy, molasses, and reserved liquids from canned vegetables.

4. Add water, cover and set the rocker.

5. Heat it till you get a steady rocking and cook for 10 minutes.

6. When ready, select the Natural Release Method and let the pressure drop naturally.

7. Stir in the vegetables and heat through.

8. Serve hot immediately.

Servings: 4

Total Cooking Time: 20 minutes

Nutrition Facts

Serving size: ¼ of a recipe (13.8 ounces)

Percent daily values based on the Reference Daily Intake (RDI) for a 2000 calorie diet.

Amount Per Serving

Calories 419

Calories From Fat (71%) 238.4

% Daily Value

Total Fat 48.6g 75%

Saturated Fat 10.3g 45%

Cholesterol 118.8mg 40%

Sodium 585.4mg 24%

Potassium 1002.4mg 29%

Total Carbohydrates 20.2g 7%

Fiber 3.5g 14%

Sugar 10.7g

Protein 25.2g 50%

Rich Minestrone Soup

Ingredients

3 lbs. tomatoes, peeled, seeded & chopped

2 cups baby spinach

1 can (11 oz.) kidney beans, drained and rinsed

2 Tbsp fresh basil, chopped

1 cup fresh corn kernels

1 zucchini, chopped

1 Tbsp olive oil

1 onion, finely chopped

2 carrots, diced

1 stalk celery, diced

4 cloves garlic, minced

2 cups water or vegetable broth

1 cup uncooked Ditaloni pasta

1 tsp Italian seasoning

1 cup grated parmesan cheese

Salt and ground black pepper to taste

Instructions

1. Select sauté and add the oil to the electric pressure cooker pot.

2. Add the onion and cook, stirring occasionally, about 4-5 minutes.

3. Add the carrots, zucchini, celery, corn, and garlic; cook about 5 minutes.

4. Add the tomatoes, water or chicken broth, pasta, spinach, Italian seasoning, and salt.

5. Lock lid in place, select high pressure and 4 minutes cook time, and start.

6. When timer beeps, turn off pressure cooker and wait 5 minutes, then do a quick pressure release.

7. Add the beans and basil. Adjust salt and pepper.

8. Serve topped with cheese.

Servings: 6

Total Cooking Time: 15 minutes

Nutrition Facts

Serving size: 1/6 of a recipe (14 ounces)

Percent daily values based on the Reference Daily Intake (RDI) for a 2000 calorie diet.

Amount Per Serving

Calories 229

Calories From Fat (36%) 83.3

% Daily Value

Total Fat 9.5g 15%

Saturated Fat 4.1g 21%

Cholesterol 18.7mg 6%

Sodium 943.3mg 39%

Potassium 877.9mg 25%

Total Carbohydrates 24.5g 8%

Fiber 5.9g 24%

Sugar 8.5g

Protein 15.1g 30%

Risotto with Portabello Mushroom

Ingredients

8 oz. portabello mushrooms, sliced

1 ½ cup risotto rice

4 cups chicken broth

4 Tbsp olive oil

4 Tbsp butter, divided

1 medium onion, diced

2 garlic cloves, minced

1 cup fresh grated Parmigiano-Reggiano cheese

Instructions

1. Pour oil and the butter into your electric pressure cooker.

2. Add garlic and onion and sauté till translucent.

3. Add portabello mushrooms and rice. Stir until rice is mixed with oil. Add chicken broth.

4. Cover with the lid and cook under high pressure for 7 minutes.

5. Release pressure with natural release method and add more butter.

6. Serve hot.

Servings: 8

Total Cooking Time: 30 minutes

Nutrition Facts

Serving size: 1/8 of a recipe (7.3 ounces)

Percent daily values based on the Reference Daily Intake (RDI) for a 2000 calorie diet.

Amount Per Serving

Calories 143.2

Calories From Fat (82%) 117.8

% Daily Value

Total Fat 13.3g 20%

Saturated Fat 4.8g 24%

Cholesterol 15.3mg 5%

Sodium 371.4mg 15%

Potassium 233.5mg 7%

Total Carbohydrates 3.3g 1%

Fiber 0.7g 3%

Sugar 1.7g

Protein 3.3g 7%

Ruddy Chicken & Pearl Onions

Ingredients

2 lbs. chicken breasts

2 cups pearl onions

3 slices pancetta

2 cups carrots, chopped

1 cup dried golden raisins

2 bay leaves

4 cloves of garlic

¼ cup balsamic vinegar

¼ red wine

½ cup water

Salt and pepper to taste

Instructions

1. Place the chicken into the bottom of your electric pressure cooker.

2. Add all remaining ingredients from the list.

3. Set the pressure valve to airtight and close the locking lid on your pressure cooker.

4. Program it to cook for 17 minutes; press start.

5. Carefully turn the pressure valve on the top to release and wait for all the steam and pressure to release.

6. The float valve will drop, allowing you to unlock the lid.

7. Carefully remove the chicken and vegetables.

8. Ladle out or pour out about half of the liquid and return it to the pressure cooker to reduce/thicken the sauce.

9. Press the start button to turn on the heating element.

10. Once the sauce is thickened to the desired consistency, carefully place the chicken back into the sauce. Set the pressure cooker to keep warm until it's ready to serve.

11. Enjoy!

Servings: 4

Total Cooking Time: 25 minutes

Nutrition Facts

Serving size: ¼ of a recipe (10.9 ounces)

Percent daily values based on the Reference Daily Intake (RDI) for a 2000 calorie diet.

Amount Per Serving

Calories 230.6

Calories From Fat (5%) 12.2

% Daily Value

Total Fat 1.4g 2%

Saturated Fat 0.3g 2%

Cholesterol 22.7mg 8%

Sodium 295mg 12%

Potassium 782mg 22%

Total Carbohydrates 38.4g 15%

Fiber 4.6g 19%

Sugar 22g

Protein 10.4g 21%

Sesame Honey Chicken

Ingredients

2 lbs. boneless skinless chicken breasts, diced

2 green onions (chopped)

1 cup diced onion

1 cup soy sauce

3 cloves garlic (minced)

¼ cup ketchup

1 cup honey

1 tsp red pepper flakes

2 Tbsp corn starch

3 Tbsp water

Sesame seeds (toasted)

2 tsp sesame oil

1 Tbsp vegetable oil

Salt and pepper

Instructions

1. In a bowl, season chicken with salt and pepper.

2. In your electric pressure cooker, add chicken, oil, onion and garlic, and cook, stirring occasionally, until onion is transparent (about 3–4 minutes).

3. Add ketchup, soy sauce, and red pepper flakes to the pressure cooking pot and stir to mix. Cook on high pressure for 3 minutes.

4. When timer beeps, turn pressure cooker off and do a quick pressure release.

5. Meanwhile, add sesame oil and honey to the pot and stir to combine.

6. In a separate pot, thaw cornstarch in water and add it to the pot. Simmer until sauce is thickened.

7. Stir in green onions. Serve hot.

Servings: 6

Total Cooking Time: 35 minutes

Nutrition Facts

Serving size: 1/6 of a recipe (9.6 ounces)

Percent daily values based on the Reference Daily Intake (RDI) for a 2000 calorie diet.

Amount Per Serving

Calories 435.1

Calories From Fat (17%) 83.2

% Daily Value

Total Fat 9.3g 14%

Saturated Fat 1.9g 10%

Cholesterol 128.5mg 43%

Sodium 935.9mg 39%

Potassium 533.2mg 15%

Total Carbohydrates 39.2g 18%

Fiber 0.7g 3%

Sugar 29.9g

Protein 48.6g 96%

Simple Rice Pudding with Raisins

Ingredients

1 cup rice

3 cups raisins

1 ½ cups water

1 tsp salt

2 cups whole milk (divided)

1 cup sugar

2 eggs

1 tsp vanilla extract

Instructions

1. Combine rice, water, and salt in your electric pressure cooker.

2. Lock the lid in place, choose high pressure and cook 3 minutes.

3. Turn off the pressure cooker and use Natural Release Method for 10 minutes.

4. Release remaining pressure with a quick pressure release.

5. Add sugar and 1 cup milk to rice in pressure cooking pot. Keep stirring to combine.

6. In a small mixing bowl, whisk eggs with remaining 1 cup milk and vanilla.

7. Pour egg mixture into pressure cooker through a fine mesh strainer.

8. Select sauté and cook, stirring continuously, until mixture starts to boil. Then turn off pressure cooker.

9. Remove the pot from the pressure cooker. Stir in raisins.

10. Let cool and serve.

Servings: 6

Total Cooking Time: 30 minutes

Nutrition Facts

Serving size: 1/6 of a recipe (8 ounces)

Percent daily values based on the Reference Daily Intake (RDI) for a 2000 calorie diet.

Amount Per Serving

Calories 309.6

Calories From Fat (10%) 31

% Daily Value

Total Fat 3.5g 5%

Saturated Fat 1.6g 8%

Cholesterol 68.5mg 23%

Sodium 163.4mg 7%

Potassium 321.8mg 9%

Total Carbohydrates 42.4g 19%

Fiber 0.8g 3%

Sugar 33.1g

Protein 7.6g 15%

Simple Spanish Risotto

Ingredients

1 cup long grain white rice

1 ¼ cup chicken broth

1 Tbsp vegetable oil

½ cup onion, diced

3 Tbsp mustard (Dijon, English, or wholegrain)

½ cup mild salsa

Salt and black ground pepper to taste

Instructions

1. Place oil in your electric pressure cooker, select sauté, and cook onions about 3 to 5 minutes.

2. Stir in rice and cook, stirring frequently, about 1 to 2 minutes.

3. Add broth, mustard and salsa. Cover and lock lid in place.

4. Select high pressure and set timer for 4 minutes. When beep sounds, wait 5 minutes and then use the Natural Release Method to release pressure.

5. When done, carefully remove lid, tilting away from you to allow steam to disperse.

6. Serve immediately.

Servings: 4

Total Cooking Time: 10 minutes

Nutrition Facts

Serving size: ¼ of a recipe (6.4 ounces)

Percent daily values based on the Reference Daily Intake (RDI) for a 2000 calorie diet.

Amount Per Serving

Calories 119.5

Calories From Fat (34%) 40.5

% Daily Value

Total Fat 4.6g 7%

Saturated Fat 0.5g 2%

Cholesterol 0mg 0%

Sodium 565.8mg 24%

Potassium 218.3mg 6%

Total Carbohydrates 16g 5%

Fiber 1.32g 5%

Sugar 2g

Protein 3.8g 8%

Scottish Apples

Ingredients

6 apples, cored

1 cup raisins

1 cup red wine

1 cup brown sugar

1 tsp cinnamon powder

Instructions

1. Add apples to your electric pressure cooker.

2. Pour in wine, raisins, sugar and cinnamon powder. Close and lock the lid of the pressure cooker. Cook for 10 minutes at high pressure.

3. When time is up, open the pressure cooker after allowing 5 to 20 minutes for the Natural Release Method.

4. Scoop apples out of the pressure cooker and serve in a small bowl with lots of cooking liquid.

Servings: 4

Total Time: 20 minutes

Nutrition Facts

Serving size: ¼ of a recipe (10.7 ounces)

Percent daily values based on the Reference Daily Intake (RDI) for a 2000 calorie diet.

Amount Per Serving

Calories 293.1

Calories From Fat (1%) 3.3

% Daily Value

Total Fat 0.4g <1%

Saturated Fat 0.06g <1%

Cholesterol 0mg 0%

Sodium 13.3mg <1%

Potassium 410.2mg 12%

Total Carbohydrates 55.3g 20%

Fiber 5.4g 21%

Sugar 44.6g

Protein 0.9g 2%

Sour Spareribs with Barbecue Sauce

Ingredients

6 lbs. spareribs

Salt and pepper

Paprika

3 tsp vegetable oil

4 onions, sliced

2 cups ketchup

1 cup vinegar

Worcestershire sauce, to taste (about 2 Tbsp)

1 tsp chili powder

1 tsp celery seeds

Instructions

1. Mix the ribs with salt, pepper and paprika. Heat in your electric pressure cooker. Add oil and brown ribs. Add sliced onions.

2. Add remaining ingredients over ribs. Close pressure cooker securely.

3. Place pressure regulator on vent pipe and cook 15 minutes at 15 pounds pressure.

4. Let pressure drop off with the Natural Release Method.

5. Serve hot.

Servings: 16

Total Cooking Time: 25 minutes

Nutrition Facts

Serving size: 1/16 of a recipe (8.4 ounces)

Percent daily values based on the Reference Daily Intake (RDI) for a 2000 calorie diet.

Amount Per Serving

Calories 424.9

Calories From Fat (70%) 367.5

% Daily Value

Total Fat 40.8g 63%

Saturated Fat 12.9g 65%

Cholesterol 136mg 45%

Sodium 367mg 15%

Potassium 565mg 16%

Total Carbohydrates 10.6g 4%

Fiber 0.7g 3%

Sugar 8g

Protein 27g 54%

Southern Short Ribs Casserole

Ingredients

2 lbs. short ribs

1 medium onion, chopped

1 large carrot

1 Tbsp brown sugar

1 can tomatoes

1 can tomato paste

3 cloves garlic

Beef stock or water

Mixed herbs

Salt and pepper to taste

Instructions

1. Mix meat with oil in a large bowl.

2. Add onion and carrot and stir with oil.

3. Add stock, crushed garlic, tomatoes and paste, mixed herbs, sugar, and salt and pepper.

4. Place all ingredients in your electric pressure cooker.

5. Lock the lid in place. Increase the stovetop heat to high and bring the cooker to high pressure. Reduce the stovetop heat to medium and cook for 30 minutes.

6. Select Natural Release Method.

7. Transfer meat and sauce to a serving plate.

Servings: 6

Total Cooking Time: 1 hour

Nutrition Facts

Serving size: 1/6 of a recipe (7.4 ounces)

Percent daily values based on the Reference Daily Intake (RDI) for a 2000 calorie diet.

Amount Per Serving

Calories 106.5

Calories From Fat (16%) 17.5

% Daily Value

Total Fat 2g 3%

Saturated Fat 0.9g 4%

Cholesterol 1.9mg <1%

Sodium 1139.6mg 47%

Potassium 564.87mg 16%

Total Carbohydrates 20g 7%

Fiber 2.8g 11%

Sugar 8.9g

Protein 14.2g 8%

Spanish Chorizo Sausages and Lentils Soup

Ingredients

¾ cup lentils

1 link chorizo sausage, chopped

2 cups tomatoes, chopped

4 cloves garlic, minced

1 cup dried vegetables mix (any)

2 bay leaves

2 cups beef broth

6 cups water

Salt and pepper to taste

Instructions

1. Place the lentils and all other ingredients from the list into your pressure cooker.

2. Shut the lid, lock it, and adjust the pressure valve to airtight.

3. Program the cook time for 15 minutes and press start.

4. When the time is up, very careful release the pressure.

5. When it is safe to open the lid, give the soup a good stir.

6. Adjust salt and pepper to taste.

7. Serve hot.

Servings: 6

Cooking Time

Total Time: 20 minutes

Nutrition Facts

Serving size: 1/6 of a recipe (16.1 ounces)

Percent daily values based on the Reference Daily Intake (RDI) for a 2000 calorie diet.

Amount Per Serving

Calories 259.4

Calories From Fat (47%) 121.5

% Daily Value

Total Fat 13.3g 20%

Saturated Fat 4.9g 25%

Cholesterol 30.2mg 10%

Sodium 838.2mg 35%

Potassium 567.2mg 16%

Total Carbohydrates 19g 6%

Fiber 8.2g 33%

Sugar 2.4g

Protein 16g 32%

Spicy Beef Chili

Ingredients

2 ½ lbs. beef chuck

1 can (11 oz.) diced tomatoes

2 Tbsp chili powder

2 tsp Spanish paprika

1 tsp chipotle chili powder

1 tsp cayenne pepper

1 tsp ground cumin

1 tsp ground black pepper

1 tsp dried oregano

4 Tbsp fresh cilantro, chopped

4 Tbsp green onions, chopped

2 Tbsp vegetable oil

1 onion, diced

4 cloves garlic

1 ½ cups water

Salt and ground black pepper to taste

Instructions

1. Heat 1 tablespoon oil in a skillet over medium-high heat.

2. Season beef with salt and black pepper; place meat within the skillet and cook till brown on all sides, 7-10 minutes.

3. Transfer to plate and set aside.

4. Heat oil over medium-low heat in the pressure cooker.

5. Stir in chili powder, paprika, cumin, black pepper, jalapeno pepper, chili powder, cayenne pepper, and oregano; cook about 2 minutes.

6. Combine diced tomatoes, beef, and water and add them.

7. Lock the lid of your pressure cooker. Increase heat to the highest level and bring to full pressure.

8. Select Natural Release Method; let the pressure drop naturally. Allow 5 to 20 minutes for this process.

9. Garnish with cilantro and onion.

Servings: 8

Total Cooking Time: 1 hour

Nutrition Facts

Serving size: 1/8 of a recipe (5.8 ounces)

Percent daily values based on the Reference Daily Intake (RDI) for a 2000 calorie diet.

Amount Per Serving

Calories 323.7

Calories From Fat (72%) 234.4

% Daily Value

Total Fat 26g 40%

Saturated Fat 9.5g 48%

Cholesterol 66.8mg 22%

Sodium 127.5mg 5%

Potassium 295.7mg 8%

Total Carbohydrates 4.8g 2%

Fiber 1.6g 6%

Sugar 1.7g

Protein 17.5g 35%

Spinach and Curried Chicken Stew

Ingredients

2 boneless chicken breasts

1 onion

1 cup dried beans

1 cup coconut milk

1 cup spinach, chopped

1 Tbsp ghee or butter

2 tsp curry powder

4 cups water

Salt

Instructions

1. Cook the chicken breasts separately.

2. Add one cup of water to the main cooking pot of your electric pressure cooker. Season the water with salt and pepper and add the chicken breasts.

3. Close the lid and turn to lock it into place. Program the pressure cooker to cook for 12 minutes. Press the start button.

4. Meanwhile, dice the onions.

5. Release the pressure by the Natural Release Method. Remove the chicken carefully with a pair of tongs, place on a plate, and set aside.

6. Discard the cooking water inside the cooking pot.

7. Place the cooking pot back into the pressure cooker. Press the start button to start the browning process.

8. Add the ghee or butter to the pot, then add the chopped onions and cook for 1–2 minutes. Add the curry powder and mix. Add the coconut milk, the beans, spinach and the remaining 3 cups of water. Stir gently.

Shut the lid and turn to lock it into place. Program the pressure cooker to cook for 30 minutes. Press the start button.

9. Let the unit drop down in pressure by itself. Serve hot.

Servings: 6

Total Cooking Time: 50 minutes

Nutrition Facts

Serving size: 1/6 of a recipe (11.7 ounces)

Percent daily values based on the Reference Daily Intake (RDI) for a 2000 calorie diet.

Amount Per Serving

Calories 200.2

Calories From Fat (43%) 86.5

% Daily Value

Total Fat 10.3g 16%

Saturated Fat 7.8g 39%

Cholesterol 24.4mg 8%

Sodium 285.7mg 12%

Potassium 402.4mg 11%

Total Carbohydrates 15.6g 5%

Fiber 3.9g 15%

Sugar 1.1g

Protein 13.5g 27%

Sweet Potato Casserole with Pecans

Ingredients

2 large sweet potatoes

1 cup brown sugar

2 Tbsp butter, melted

1 tsp vanilla

1 tsp ground cinnamon

1/8 tsp ground nutmeg

1 egg

2 Tbsp heavy cream

Topping

1 Tbsp butter (melted)

3 Tbsp brown sugar

1 Tbsp flour

1/3 cup pecans (chopped)

Instructions

1. Peel and cut sweet potatoes in half lengthwise and then cut into 1-inch slices.

2. Place a steamer basket in your electric pressure cooker pot.

3. Pour in 1 cup water and sliced potatoes. Lock lid in place and choose high pressure for 8 minutes.

4. When timer beeps, turn off pressure cooker and quickly release pressure. When the pressure is released, carefully take out the lid.

5. Place sweet potatoes in a mixing bowl and add brown sugar, vanilla, butter, cinnamon, and nutmeg. Beat with an electric mixer until smooth.

6. Add egg and cream. Blend well. Pour into greased casserole dish.

7. Whisk together butter, brown sugar, flour and nuts with a fork; scatter over top of casserole.

8. Place the stand in the pressure cooker pot. Add 1 cup water.

9. Lock lid in place and cook on high pressure for 15 minutes.

10. Serve hot.

Servings: 6

Total Cooking Time: 25 minutes

Nutrition Facts

Serving size: 1/6 of a recipe (4.9 ounces)

Percent daily values based on the Reference Daily Intake (RDI) for a 2000 calorie diet.

Amount Per Serving

Calories 235.9

Calories From Fat (44%) 102.6

% Daily Value

Total Fat 11.9g 18%

Saturated Fat 4.9g 24%

Cholesterol 49.7mg 17%

Sodium 22.2mg <1%

Potassium 83.5mg 2%

Total Carbohydrates 32.1g 11%

Fiber 0.8g 3%

Sugar 28g

Protein 1.9g 4%

Tangy Pumpkin Soup

Ingredients

1 Tbsp butter

1 butternut pumpkin

1 potato, diced

2 green onions, chopped

1 apple, peeled, cored and grated

3 cups chicken stock

Curry powder

Salt and black pepper to taste

4 bay leaves

2 cups milk

Instructions

1. Melt butter in your electric pressure cooker.

2. Add pumpkin chunks, onion, potato and a pinch of curry powder.

3. Cook over low heat for 2–3 minutes, stirring occasionally.

4. Add the chicken stock, black pepper and bay leaves.

5. Secure the lid and bring to pressure. Cook for 5 minutes.

6. Release pressure using the Natural Release Method.

7. Stir in the grated apple and cook uncovered for 10 minutes, stirring occasionally.

8. Remove the bay leaves.

9. Transfer the soup to a blender, add the milk and process until soup is creamy.

10. Serve warm.

Servings: 8

Preparation Time: 25 minutes

Nutrition Facts

Serving size: 1/8 of a recipe (10.5 ounces)

Percent daily values based on the Reference Daily Intake (RDI) for a 2000 calorie diet.

Amount Per Serving

Calories 116.2

Calories From Fat (26%) 29.7

% Daily Value

Total Fat 3.3g 5%

Saturated Fat 1.9g 9%

Cholesterol 8.7mg 3%

Sodium 307.8mg 13%

Potassium 578.5mg 17%

Total Carbohydrates 17.4g 6%

Fiber 1.8g 7%

Sugar 7.7g

Protein 5.4g 11%

Tapioca Coconut Pudding

Ingredients

½ cup small-pearl tapioca

½ cup coconut milk

½ cup coconut sugar

2 egg yolks

1 ½ cups water

½ tsp vanilla extract

¼ tsp salt

Instructions

1. Add tapioca and water to your electric pressure cooker; stir well.

2. Lock the lid in place; select high pressure and 6 minutes cook time.

3. When ready, use the Natural Release Method.

4. Whisk coconut sugar and salt into tapioca in pressure cooking pot.

5. Whisk egg yolks with milk. Pour through a fine mesh strainer into pressure cooking pot.

6. Select sauté and cook, stirring constantly, until mixture just starts to boil.

7. Turn off pressure cooker and remove pressure cooking pot. Stir in vanilla.

8. Let cool, pour in serving dishes and serve.

Servings: 4

Total Time: 15 minutes

Nutrition Facts

Serving size: ¼ of a recipe (6.1 ounces)

Percent daily values based on the Reference Daily Intake (RDI) for a 2000 calorie diet.

Amount Per Serving

Calories 253.6

Calories From Fat (28%) 72

% Daily Value

Total Fat 8.4g 13%

Saturated Fat 6.3g 32%

Cholesterol 90mg 30%

Sodium 156mg 7%

Potassium 83mg 2%

Total Carbohydrates 43.9g 15%

Fiber 0.2g <1%

Sugar 25.7g

Protein 1.9g 4%

White Bean Soup with Squash and Chard

Ingredients

16 oz. dried white beans

2 cups butternut squash (diced)

4 cups Swiss chard leaves

8 cups chicken stock

1 large onion (chopped)

3 carrots (chopped)

3 stalks celery (chopped)

4 sprigs fresh rosemary

1 Tbsp olive oil

1 tsp fresh rosemary (chopped)

4 garlic cloves (sliced),

1 cup chicken stock

1 cup sour cream

Salt, pepper

1 cup croutons

Instructions

1. Heat oil in pressure cooker and sauté celery and onion until soft.

2. Add white beans, rosemary sprigs, chicken stock and pepper.

3. Bring the pressure to 15 and cook it for 35 minutes.

4. Using the quick release cold water method, open the lid and add butternut squash, minced rosemary, garlic, and salt & pepper to taste.

5. Replace lid and cook for 10 additional minutes before using the Natural Release Method.

6. Test beans to ensure they're completely soft.

7. Take out rosemary stems. Adjust salt and pepper to taste.

8. Stir in chard greens just before serving.

9. Serve with a dollop of sour cream and croutons.

Servings: 6

Total Time: 1 hour and 20 minutes

Nutrition Facts

Serving size: 1/6 of a recipe (13.8 ounces)

Percent daily values based on the Reference Daily Intake (RDI) for a 2000 calorie diet.

Amount Per Serving

Calories 345.1

Calories From Fat (19%) 83.8

% Daily Value

Total Fat 9.4g 14%

Saturated Fat 3.4g 17%

Cholesterol 9.9mg 3%

Sodium 1264.3mg 53%

Potassium 1459.1mg 48%

Total Carbohydrates 44.8g 22%

Fiber 15.1g 60%

Sugar 6.2g

Protein 27.7g 55%

www.ingramcontent.com/pod-product-compliance
Lightning Source LLC
Chambersburg PA
CBHW070059030426
42335CB00016B/1945